The Anaemic Leukaemic
A Message of Hope

John Fee

authorHOUSE®

AuthorHouse™ UK Ltd.
500 Avebury Boulevard
Central Milton Keynes, MK9 2BE
www.authorhouse.co.uk
Phone: 08001974150

First published by AuthorHouse 8/16/2010

ISBN: 978-1-4520-3899-5 (sc)

This book is printed on acid-free paper.

Contents

Part Two - A Simple Man's Guide to Cancer, The Universe and Everything

Preface

Having faced death with a diagnosis of Leukaemia what else was there left in the world for me to fear? This was a time to reflect on life, why was I here in this body at this time? Why was I experiencing this suffering ? What was I being shown? How many more questions can there possibly be ?

My belief system includes the fact that all we experience in life we do so for a reason, this includes disease and illness. For me, cancer took me out of the classic stressful job scenario and gave me time out to reflect on where I go from here. It also gave me a lesson in trust, or what some people refer to as faith, trusting all would be well and that I would be looked after whatever the outcome. Life threatening illness, unemployed, house up for sale in a recession, in debt……..the only way was upwards ! I was forced to live life in the moment, after all that is all there is in reality. Ultimately though, I am healed, this through a combination of Western orthodox medicine and complementary and alternative therapies which have helped me to recover from the dreaded 'Chemo'! I am a survivor, here is my tale and I share with you what I have learnt along the somewhat rocky path that has been my journey through cancer.

The aim of this book is twofold. Firstly I wish to show you that yes, unbelievable as it may sound, there is humour in the world of cancer ! What I experienced was a somewhat brutal regime which has a deep physical and psychological impact on one's self. There were some ridiculous and worryingly funny scenarios however, which I wish to share with you. If you are experiencing cancer I hope to bring you some light relief from the suffering. If you have never had cancer I hope that situation remains, ultimately I hope I can allay some of the fears and reduce some of the stigma which still surrounds the 'Big C'.

In the Second half of the book I wish to share with you what I have learnt about the mystery that is cancer. I am an inquisitive soul, some would say nosey, and I wanted to find out what did cause my cancer. I did not believe the 'there is no known cause' statement which all the literature on leukaemia suggested. In answering this I went on a journey of discovery that led me to develop a simple model for those who are serious about healing themselves. I have examined what cancer is, it's growing prevalence and how we treat it in this country and elsewhere. The concept of miraculous or spontaneous remissions appears to be largely ignored by the medical profession but was of major interest to me. I share with you what I found along with what worked for me, which, I acknowledge will not automatically work for you for we are, after all, unique and individual beings. The model I have created does give individuals a framework for true healing to begin to take place. How you choose to get that healing is your choice.

There are numerous conspiracy theorists who would advocate that there are no vast profits to be had in complementary medicine and as such they are not allowed to compete with the pharmaceutical companies who make billions of pounds profit each year. Having said that, without such drugs as developed by said pharmaceutical giants, I would not be sat sitting typing this! The main problem at this moment in time is that individuals generally have to pay for complementary therapies themselves. The increase in usage of such therapies, however means that we appear to be beginning to take control of our own health. The more these therapies are used, the nearer we are to them becoming more mainstream and incorporated as part of routine treatments, whether the medical profession views them as quackery or not!

Surprisingly, there were positives to come out of this experience. As Lance Armstrong, the world famous cyclist and seven times winner of the Tour de France states in his book "*It's Not About the Bike*" (known to us cancer survivors simply as 'The Book'), cancer was the best thing that happened to him. For me, it showed me a world full of love, kindness, empathy and practical support along with an increased sense of community. A world very different from that portrayed by the mass media. Cancer gave me the nudge I needed to fulfil my life purpose and get on living life with joy and gratitude instead of being miserable with my lot and feeling I was a victim. Sometimes we need to experience the really dark times in our life in order for us to recognise what truly amazing beings we are and to recognise the Light.

I do not want this to be seen merely as an opportunity to criticise the current approaches to cancer within the health service, after all without this current system I would probably have been scattered on the Lakeland fells by now! I am no guru, in fact the last time I attempted the lotus position it ended in a near hospital admission and an introduction to daily application of copious amounts of liniment along with a John Wayne walk for a few weeks. What I have written comes from the heart. I have no vested interest other than seeking to empower others to make informed choices on their health. Please see this as an opportunity to look at how we as human beings can move things forward for the benefit of us all. We can look both within ourselves and at the system to improve our healthcare in order that it become truly holistic and subsequently successful. The increasing mortality rate of cancer sufferers would surely suggest that the current system we use isn't working that well! Maybe, together, we can create a world where cancer is a thing of the past. Just imagine, a world without cancer......

Acknowledgements

From the bottom of my heart, thank you to those who walked alongside me during my toughest challenge yet and have proved the power of love:-

Sandra my beloved soul mate who suffered as I did, Mum & Dad, Janice & Mike, Caitlin & Younger (the text demons), David & Judith (for the free computer which made life so much easier), Colin & Dorothy, June & Ken, Vanessa & John, Fiona & Andrew, Allan & Sue, Lynne & Chris, Malcolm, Brian & Bev, Karen & Dave, Nigel & Jacqui, Gerard, Dorothy & Matt, Glyn, Chris & Anne, Richard & Betty, Lynn & John, Denise & John, Elaine & David (the Computer Supremo), Kevin, Rowena, Denise & Derek, Carolyn & Alan, Glyn & Jan, Stuart & Tony, Teresa, Janet, Len & Tracy, Helen, Christine, Lesa, Katie & Simon, Neil & Ang, John & Pauline, Jane & Joyce, Elizabeth, Stephen, Stuart & Tony, Rob & Rich. All at The Glenmore Trust, Carlisle who helped support Sandra through this with tenderness, kindness and empathy. All those kindly people in our lives too numerous to mention, you know who you are!

Special thanks to those who helped me stay:

Vernon & Sue: For easing our financial burdens, thank you.
Anne Ward: for directing your amazing healing powers in my direction with love.
Jan Ford-Batey: The best Naturopath in the whole wide world!
Ray Balmain: The most down to earth enlightened being I know, thanks for all the hidden healings.

Joe & Sue: For showing me what courage really is.

Briony Stott: For your help in ridding me of years of baggage

Professor Graham Jackson, Dr Hugh O'Brien, The staff of Ward 8, RVI, Newcastle & Larch D Ward , Cumberland Infirmary, Carlisle : Thank you for sharing your amazing knowledge and skills with me during my cancer journey, you are amazing people.

All Blood Donors: You saved my life!

Carol Charlton: A wonderful Social Worker who eased the pressures

Dr Nair: For seeing me through the dark days with compassion.

All those people that don't know me but yet still prayed for me, especially at Caldbeck Methodist Chapel. Prayer really works!

Finally, grateful thanks to my agent Darin Jewell of Inspira Group, who had faith in me and the book and whose drive and enthusiasm made all this possible.

Dedicated to my soul mate Sandra, who suffered as much, if not more than I did, but helped me just by being there when it really mattered. We made it!!

Part One

My Journey Through Cancer

"May it be an evening star shines down on you,
  May it be when darkness falls, your heart be true"

Enya

Chapter One

This Is Me!

The Arrival

"Oh What a Night, Late December Back in '63………..". Well it was the 16th to be precise, and more like afternoon, 2.45pm at Batley Maternity Home when I decided to enter the world. 7 lbs 12 ozs of pink (more likely blue as it was mid-winter and there wasn't much in the way of heating back then) joy and fun on legs. Where all that joy and fun disappeared to is a mystery although I have to say it's starting to re-emerge now thankfully. So, a little brother for Janice who was 4, the Fee family was complete.

If I was to have written an autobiography, I suppose it could have been marketed as "The cure for Insomniacs" or "If you thought your life was dull wait till you read about this guy…". What I am trying to say is that my life has up to this point not exactly been the most exciting you will ever read about, just call me Mr Ordinary. I have, it must be said, brought others joy and laughter along the way, this usually as a result of my own misfortune or accident proneness and I now look upon the latter as a gift.

Dad worked for a bank and in those days was moved every 2-3 years to gain experience in different aspects of banking as it was a knowledgeable and skilful occupation in the days before

"Computer Says No" technology. So from Batley we moved to Northumberland then back to Rastrick, West Yorkshire (one half of the world famous brass band) and then when I was 10 we moved "down South" to Nottingham. I felt like the equivalent of a young Michael Palin ! Where to next….

School Daze

I arrived at my new school in Nottingham with a heavy Yorkshire accent which made Geoffrey Boycott sound as though he spoke the Queens English. I also made somewhat of an impact in the Midlands by sporting short trousers, as they did in Yorkshire. Big mistake ! Infants, seemingly in Nottingham wore long trousers. Spot the new kid, Yorkshire accent, short trousers, it is what psychologists call character building or more likely the beginnings of some deep rooted anxiety disorder ! I call it pre-long trouser disorder (PLTD). However, with a bit of bribery and corruption, always a better option than outright violence I always think, I was accepted, especially when I was found to be reasonable at football.

School never really appealed. I gained 7 O' levels, stayed on at sixth form and realised that I had reached my educational zenith leaving with a couple of low graded A' levels. Hardly surprising that, as I spent the majority of my sixth form days playing snooker and tennis and generally lazing. Despite this admission I doubt whether I would have achieved more had I received one to one tuition. My memory has always let me down and in a system that tested memory I was always onto a loser so to speak.

Of Cash Tins and Ink Pads

So, I joined the world of paid employment working for a rival bank to dad's, this so I could prove I got the job on my own merit and not under the old nepotism ploy ! A new suit and a haircut and off I went, a nervous bag of hormonal teenager into the world of high finance. My tendency towards being accident prone unfortunately went along with me and I will share with you an example to give you a flavour of my leaning towards disasterism in those heady days of banking.....

I spent the first few weeks in the bank acquiring the skills and knowledge to enable me to become a cashier and this particular Monday morning I was going solo. For a pimply self conscious teenager this was the equivalent of the first flight as a pilot without the instructor there. I arrived well in time for the nine o'clock start to get my till prepared for the nine thirty opening. The counters were wooden and were about chest height and each cashier had a tall stool on which to sit (a bit like Dave Allen for those that are old enough to remember him but without the cigarettes and whisky). I preferred to stand to get my till ready and had my metal cash box on top of the counter to count and check all the cash I was taking control of. There was a lot of change on this till and this along with phone calls to answer meant I was running late and still had the cash tin on top of the counter as the branch was opened and the customers began to pour in.

Trembling I closed the cash tin, locked it and lifted it off the counter to drop it underneath the counter on the floor where it was usually stored. On getting back up it was then I realised I had trapped my nice new tie in the tin and due to the tin being the equivalent to a concrete block in weight ,I was now well and truly stuck. The keys were on top of the counter where a now curious queue of customers waited with baited breath to see the ghost like new boy 'Mr Fee'. I needed the keys and so reached up onto the counter, and being unable to see I had to locate them by feel. Unfortunately my hand firstly located the freshly inked pad and after much rummaging found the jewel in the crown, the said keys. By this time the adrenaline was in full flow, like a formula one driver when the lights turn green, I was pumping ! The keys unlocked me from my cash tin shackle and I adjusted my tie with my right hand, which, on rising, I now realised was the same hand that had warmly greeted the ink pad just moments before. I stood up, red faced due to a complicated mixture of embarrassment and partial strangulation with black hand and now hand imprinted tie. "Are you alright ?" the first lady customer asked quizzically. "Perfectly", I responded.

There were other similar disastrous events such as triggering the alarm system at a major bank in Manchester whilst in the middle of taking a banking exam after hours. I was doing well until the armed police arrived…..No-one had mentioned the alarm buttons under the counter where I was fiddling trying to understand which language the exam paper was in. I failed needless to say and would have done without the interruption.

In terms of my list of personal calamities, I do have a favourite, this in the form of my briefcase becoming trapped in the door of the bus as I was getting off. The driver, being unaware, allegedly, set off with me running alongside until the bus stopped at some traffic lights some 100m up the road. Here I was able to alert said driver of my plight. The presence of a wry grin suggested this was obviously a common ploy, probably in the Bus Drivers Manual Vol 4 : "Commuters – Potential Entertainment for You and Your Passengers". "Sorry mate" was the response. Since when do 'mates' do things like that to each other ? Still, it reminds me of those heady days before the well known double act of Health & Safety arrived on the scene…..

Human Remains

By now you will have a slight inkling as to why my banking career never really left the launch pad, or should that be ink pad ! I was still in the metaphorical dressing room when I left the organisation 7 years later to join British Rail, changing career to work in personnel or HR (Human Resources) as it fashionably became. There were some unkind quarters who used to refer to us as the Human Remains Department. There were times when I have to admit that the office did rather resemble a collection of the living dead, myself included.

My British Rail career took off, surprisingly. Maybe the phrase "Promoting people to the level of their incompetence" applied to me in this case. I reached the heights of lower management. I met some lovely people, my wife and soul mate Sandra being the loveliest of all. There was a real sense of family about the railway as it was then. It was unfortunate to see this culture eroded as the great railway sell off known as privatisation took place. Colleagues suddenly found themselves on the payroll of opposing companies and what were often solid friendships became sorely tested as a different stressful culture came to prevail. Time for me to depart.....

A Closet Carer

I had always had a leaning towards caring for others which manifested in a number of ways. There were numerous trips North to Barrow-In-Furness to help care for ageing and poorly grandparents, there was a tendency to end up looking after the more elderly customers in the bank and there was a leaning towards the welfare side of personnel management. Thus I left my management position within the company I had ended up at post privatisation on the railway network and became...
.........a student nurse. A mature student nurse. After my first day at the University of Nottingham, School of Nursing and Midwifery, I discovered I was a *very* mature student nurse. I was old enough to be the father of the majority of my intake.

Three years raced past and I qualified gaining my diploma in Mental Health Nursing. Sandra and I had always wanted to move North, and this we did on completion of my training . I managed to get a job on a ward which cared for older people with various types of dementia. If this book is successful there is potential for a follow up under the title "Diaries of a Psychiatric Nurse" by John Fee aged 45 ¾ but feeling 87 ! The following years saw me progress to the position of Community Psychiatric Nurse again working with older people out in the wilds of rural Cumbria. It was whilst undertaking this role that it all started to go sadly wrong.........

Stress and Strain

I had always carried with me a degree of anxiety along with a need to keep the peace and please others plus a hefty chunk of the "Be perfect" driver to quote a bit of psychobabble. Some baggage to carry around ! From an employers perspective I was quite a find as I would strive to achieve the utmost quality in whatever I did. For me though, this would take its toll particularly in the latter years where the litigious society impacted greatly on the health service in the form of increased bureaucracy and potentially less patient contact for nurses across the service as a result. To do both paperwork and maintain maximum contact with an ever increasing caseload in the community which included some seriously unwell people began to make its mark on my physical wellbeing.

The Itch You Can't Scratch

The more astute of you will have realised that the mood has changed over the past few paragraphs to that of a more serious note. On reflection that is probably because it brings back over two years of suffering. It wasn't much fun back then to be truthful. I'm not your typical leukaemic according to the literature. My symptoms developed gradually to start with. Initially I began to experience itching over my torso, back, arms and legs after having a bath or shower. Thinking that this was down to how I used to rub myself dry quite vigorously (calm down dear) I began to gently pat myself dry. The symptoms began to escalate and I noticed that heat made the itching worse so I took to having luke warm showers, baths were a no go area. Luke warm showers in mid-winter was grim. I began to experience night sweats and can now empathise with women experiencing them as part of the menopause. I would wake up with the duvet soaking and then the itching would start having been triggered by the heat. I would have to get up and to cope with the severe agitation the itching caused would either go out for a walk in the middle of the night or pace the floor of the lounge for 2-3 hours until the itching went off. Scratching made it worse in case you're wondering.

The other main symptom I experienced was lethargy or tiredness. Having been fit and active, running and walking, I found walking short distances left me bushed and the running was definitely out of bounds. I started taking Antihistamine tablets prescribed by my GP, these to try and combat the itching. However, they only made me more tired and with hindsight I shouldn't have been driving which I was until April 2008 when said GP duly signed me off work. Other little symptoms began to appear, such as regular mouth ulcers and the fungal infection of my nails began to spread to other parts of my body.

I was referred to see a Dr O'Brien at the Cumberland Infirmary, a Consultant Haematologist, to see what he would make of me. After blood tests and a bone marrow biopsy (ouch) I was shown to have a "low grade Neutropaenia" which meant that my immune system was compromised but no underlying cause was found as to why this should be. All were flummoxed, myself included. I consulted a naturopath who tested me using kinesiology and put me on a diet and supplements to deal with my fungal infection and to help my thyroid and adrenal systems which were on the verge of resigning !

As if all that was not enough I was now allergic to house dust mites, sheep and livestock and probably life with hindsight.

Ending It All

By this time I was not on the top of anyone's list for invites to parties, come to think of it I wasn't on the list at all. My mood had plummeted and if I had been offered a pill to end it all whilst I was pacing the floor at 3am I would have taken it, no problem. I had had enough. It was no joke getting up every day knowing that there was a day of suffering ahead. I was a pathetic, apathetic specimen. Time to stop the bus and get off (minus briefcase).

A Glimmer of Hope

My GP was very understanding and things started to improve. The symptoms grew less severe, probably a combination of less stress out of work and the remedies I was taking. I began to feel better and accepted that maybe it was all related to stress. After much discussion with Sandra we decided my nursing career, albeit short and sweet was over. My GP did state that "Most of the good nurses leave" which I took as a compliment.

I applied for and got a part time position as an advocate for people with learning difficulties and will always be grateful and yet surprised for them employing me, maybe I was the only one who turned up ! After two weeks, however, I verbally resigned after finding the organisation quite extreme in its outlook. I agreed to stay until they found a replacement. Financially things were going to get tough. We put the house up for sale, this appearing to be the only solution apart from a lottery win.

The Feinting Hitler

It was at this time I began to get sores appearing on my face. One appeared under my nose and lasted for three weeks, my identity photo taken at this time makes me look like Hitler. A different GP to my own diagnosed folliculitis and prescribed a course of antibiotics which helped but I then ended up with oral thrush (a nasty ailment which can result in ulcerations in the mouth). The folliculitis returned and a stronger course of antibiotics resulted in severe oral thrush, I was unable to eat solid food for two weeks and was in tremendous pain. I was prescribed treatment for the thrush and strong painkillers. I hope you're managing to keep up with all this and haven't put the book on the "read if there's nowt else available" pile or still worse out for the latest charity "We need your bric-a-brac" plastic bag – collection day is Thursday by the way.

It was amidst all this that I passed out in the bathroom one morning at 6am on the way to taking the dog for a walk. Sandra, bless her, had just been on her First Aid course at work so I came round with my right foot behind my left ear in the recovery position. We thought that I'd overdosed on Co-Codamol, a fairly strong painkiller and so I returned to bed and phoned in sick. I returned to work a few days later still struggling to eat and went back to see the GP I had been seeing about all this face and mouth carry on. She decided on more medication for the thrush and a blood test. Oh dear.

D-Day Looms

The evening following having the blood test I received a call from the head of the Surgery asking us both to go in straight away. This we duly did and were told that the blood results were not good and that Dr O'Brien the Consultant Haematologist wanted to see us both at the Infirmary at 9am in the morning and "Take an overnight bag as you'll be spending a few days in hospital…." Crikey, I've got no jamas, what do I wear except for a smile ?

Chapter Two

I Become A Leukaemic !

The Journey Continues – Diagnosis or D-Day

So there we were, Sandra and I, post surgery discussion. As humans we have an amazing capacity to cope, in my case it was through convincing myself and others, Sandra, mum and dad, that it was some problem with my immune system which obviously needed some further investigations hence the hospital stay. Having put that in a box file within my mind I could concentrate on the really important things such as 'what do I do about pyjamas?' talk about fiddling while Rome burns, just call me Nero!

Surprisingly I slept well that night. We had arranged for doggy day care for Toby, our faithful companion, with mum and dad, something he was used to on a regular basis and so we dropped him off on the way to the Cumberland Infirmary at Carlisle to see Dr Hugh O'Brien, Consultant Haematologist. Having seen him before for a bone marrow biopsy in April at least I knew he was personable and approachable. As soon as we arrived he ushered us in to one of his consulting rooms and closed the door – in a few months time I would know this to be a bad sign. "Right John, you've got Leukaemia. You're booked in at Newcastle RVI under Professor Graham Jackson. They have a Centre of Excellence over there and you're in good hands with Graham ...."

The rest I have to admit to losing. I vaguely remember muttering "I have leukaemia" more as an affirmation than a question. Dr O'Brien referred to the bone marrow in April stating that he'd sent it to a colleague for a second opinion but it was inconclusive at that time. "They will take another biopsy in Newcastle to confirm diagnosis, do you know how to get there?"

Thereafter followed a debate between Sandra and I as to whether we get the train or drive. I was in no state to drive. Dr O'Brien left to get us train times and by his return we'd decided to drive. My world was starting to collapse. I am a lousy passenger and now had to rely on Sandra, my faithful soul mate, who had only driven on a motorway a few times! At times of crisis such as these people can draw on their hidden strengths and surprise themselves and others. Sandra certainly girded up her loins on this occasion. Dr O'Brien drew us a map of the route from the outskirts of Newcastle to the RVI – Royal Victoria Infirmary – a place I was to get to know intimately. We left after 15 minutes in the hospital and ventured outside. It was pouring down and blowing a gale. As I went to give our parking ticket to the person taking our spot Dr O'Brien's map blew out of the car and disappeared over the horizon – Brilliant. There appeared, however, a ray of sunshine and a rainbow – maybe this was a sign not to give up hope.

So, here I was, left to focus on guiding Sandra to Newcastle and desperately trying to find a box file in my mind to put this leukaemia thing. I decided it maybe needed a filing cabinet as it kept spilling out and resulting in tears and the need to find a toilet!

The Crying Twins

We decided to stop at Hexham, our usual stop whenever we head over to the North East, usually for holidays and happy times. I suggested getting something to eat and we found a café which had been vegetarian when we last used it a few years ago. We ordered some soup and a roll. Sandra managed to loosen her hands from the 'gripping the wheel' pose to pick up her spoon and off we went. It was then that the tears started, I triggered Sandra and we both sat there blubbing. The waiter obviously thought we were distraught over the soup but decided he didn't do counselling and left us alone. Other people in the café suddenly struck up conversations where silence had reigned or busily began eating or drinking whatever was available. This was Britain, come on chaps, keep that upper lip stiffened, please.

Thus, with a plentiful supply of café napkins for tissues we rallied ourselves and got the soup, potato and leek, as I recall, down our necks. My mindset now was thus akin to a last day of freedom (who says I lack insight). To that end I ordered a slab of chocolate cake and went for it in such a way as to make Sandra appear to be a carer for the day helping someone integrate back into society, or merely be present in 'the community'. So that was my last supper, so to speak. We headed back to the car, the sun appeared after rain and lo and behold another rainbow. Definitely some sort of signage going on here ....

The Emotional Rollercoaster

Having been out of a city for some eight years since we left Nottingham all we needed was the smock and pitchfork and the look of a country bumpkin would have been complete. Our first major obstacle was the huge roundabout on the outskirts of Newcastle. I would love to meet the designer of such vast pieces of highway infrastructure. I have visions of it being an apprentice civil engineering student, being given the task by his superiors. The roundabout in question starts well with each of the fifty lanes as you approach being labelled on the road as to where they will take you, so far so good for our apprentice friend, who unbeknown to the innocent driver is lulling said driver in to a false sense of security. Once on the roundabout the lane you thought you were following merges with twenty others resulting in much horn usage and gesturing by the locals, somewhat reminiscent of driving in Cairo where the first rule of driving is 'There are no rules'. I guess it was a Friday afternoon job in the world of highway planning..... Sandra did brilliantly under the circumstances and we headed off in the right direction towards the City Centre.

Parking was a nightmare, Sandra was getting stressed so I took over the driving and we eventually found a multi-storey car park run by Dick Turpin Associates. The record charge for us was over £6 for about half a day. I informed Sandra that she may as well bring the deeds to the house if she were going to visit overnight! So, the car was parked, overnight bag in hand we began the search for Ward 8. It is no exaggeration to say it was the most distant point from the car park, a sled and a team of huskies would have been more appropriate than legs that were getting increasingly wobbly due to the increasing by the minute anaemia and subsequent lack of energy.

We arrived both exhausted, physically and mentally, onto Ward 8. This was to be home for the next 4-5 weeks. We were met immediately by one of the doctors and ushered into a consulting room to see Professor Jackson who introduced himself as Graham and was a very approachable and warm person. He went on to explain I had Acute Myeloid Leukaemia or 'AML'. Why do we have to abbreviate everything? I suppose it does make it sound less life threatening, 'AML', sounded quite catchy, I liked it. I imagined all the country's professors getting together – now look here chaps, we can't call this thing Acute Myeloid Leukaemia, it sounds too much of a mouthful and sounds a bit too serious – any suggestions? 'How about just AML?' Yes, like it, it's got style, it's punchy and rolls off the tongue. All agreed – good show!

Professor Jackson went on to explain about what would happen. I would need to have a bone marrow biopsy to confirm diagnosis and would then commence chemotherapy straight away. Did I have any siblings as a bone marrow transplant may be part of the treatment? I explained I had an older sister, Janice and they would arrange to have her blood analysed to see if she was a match, if she agreed that is, which she did and she was (a perfect match that is).

At least in Professor Jackson I had someone who is and presented as an expert in his field who would look me in the eye and instil positive feelings. This fellow of the human race clearly understood people, observing him over the following months I realised how blessed we all were to have him on our side. He altered his approach seamlessly depending upon the needs of that individual. Some clearly were in fear and didn't want to know anything – Graham would leave them feeling good about things even where situations appeared bleak for the casual observer. "We are here to get you into remission, we don't talk about cure at this stage ………" Later conversations showed he could have expanded on this to say you've not got long to live. My life was saved by Professor Jackson, his team of equally dedicated Consultants and doctors and nursing staff. The scientists who developed the chemotherapy must also be mentioned. I did get to remission after each treatment, the positive approach worked in my case, I had immediate trust in this man who looked into my soul on that first meeting.

Up to this point I had adopted the stiff upper lip 'I can cope with whatever you throw at me type' person. Underneath and within was a different, quivering beast altogether! We were shown to my room ! I had my own cubicle complete with TV and sink etc. I put my energies into the practical things such as unpacking my 'overnight' bag which seemed pretty inadequate considering the lengthy sentence I had received. My thoughts turned to Sandra and her pending solo adventure in the form of the return journey to Wigton. This was mid-winter, it would be dark at 4pm at the latest, it was now 2pm. We agreed after much tears she should leave now to get back in some daylight. I put on my acting head and reassured her that I would be fine – she had begun the equally daunting role of cancer sufferer's carer. On her return home, which took an interesting scenic diversion over the Tyne Bridge and through

Gateshead, Sandra began the unenviable task of ringing up relatives and friends with the news and the subsequent emotional rollercoaster that this process would involve with each phone call.

So, Sandra departed to continue her white knuckle liaison with big roundabouts and I sat contemplating. Catherine, the Haematology Nurse Specialist paid me a visit armed with pamphlets and information primarily to introduce herself and to have a chat to see if I had any questions about things. Shortly into the conversation she asked me if I had any children, on responding that we didn't she then opted to hit the button marked "Press for emotional release – Danger stand well clear " by asking whether I had any pets. "We've got a dog" I blubbed, the tears streaming down as I realised I would be away from our dear canine companion for at least a month. How would he deal with it all ? I had never been away from him since we got him from the Eden Animal Rescue some 4 years ago.

Catherine's role is a difficult one but is also invaluable. Here was a person you could ask to see whenever you wanted and who would provide a more informal link between you and the Consultants and provide information and support when it was needed. The difficult side to her role is dealing with the psychological needs of those in her care which can often be hidden and complex. There would be times, probably on a daily basis where she is supporting people for whom treatment has failed to address their illness.

I was left with a fistful of pamphlets as opposed to dollars. Truth be told I was never further from the macho character with no name played by Clint Eastwood, here was a jellified wreck trying to appear to the outside world as though everything was under control. Fat chance! The pamphlets turned out to be very informative about 'AML' (still catchy isn't it) its' treatment and other sources of information and support. They did help to quell the "Oh my God I'm going to die !" thought which unnervingly kept popping in. I was offered a referral to Social Services which I gratefully accepted, after all there were still the practical issues to deal with such as the lack of income, the mortgage etc.... Here I was, life threatening illness, no job for the first time since leaving school and our beloved house up for sale in the worst recession since the dawn of man according to the press. I needed help and fast!

Choice, What Choice?

The initial meeting with Professor Jackson brought home the gravity of the situation. I was basically given a choice, accept treatment or die, although it was phrased slightly better than that. It was however, that simple. I had always boasted in the past that I would refuse chemotherapy if it were me in that situation when looking at people with cancer. I saw it as a brutal way of treating people. Here I was though, having to eat humble pie and accept that there was no alternative treatment I could afford that would bring me back from the brink of death where I now stood quivering, or more likely leaning with support! The guy following me about dressed in black and banging his scythe into the furniture was becoming a serious threat. I had to face this character called Death, look into his (why is it a he?) perceived deep and soulless eyes and decide whether I was to go with him or stay and face the music. Those eyes weren't those of a monster, they were soft and full of hope and love, the black cloak was cast aside to reveal angelic white. Death was not to fear, there is life beyond, this I know.

Choose Life.

I decided I was to stay and battle at an early stage. Here I was being given an opportunity. I was being taken out of the day to day reality of work, mortgages and all the associated stress. I was being closeted from all this and allowed time and space to rest without a care. This in itself was a blessing and a relief in its own way. Together with the overwhelming support from family, friends, neighbours and from quarters unlooked for, these things enforced the fact that the world is indeed full of love, and is a very different animal from that portrayed by the media on a daily basis who would have us believe that violence, hatred and anger abound. My sister, Janice sent me a parcel filled with creature comforts including a picture of Toby our dog which I duly set up on my bedside cabinet after more tears. I had made my mark and was beginning to settle in. There would be times though when I thought that the decision to stay and battle through was highly delusional !

The Bank with Strange Deposits

One slight disadvantage for the newly diagnosed leukaemic is the fact that the treatment can lead to "*Temporary or permanent*" infertility. For me this did not pose a major problem, being one of those strange types that has never felt the urge to enter the world of fatherhood – looking after a canine companion is as far as I wish to go in terms of responsibility for others! However, part of the diagnosis 'chat', and I use the term lightly as it was a somewhat one sided conversation due to me being a quivering, befuddled wreck, is to give the apprentice leukaemic the chance to either store sperm (for men, obviously) or more rarely, a woman's eggs or fertilised eggs (embryos). Due to the nature of the illness however, time may be a limiting factor as treatment more often than not has to commence as soon as possible, leaving little time for such procedures.

During later periods of incapacity I was left with time to ponder the enigma that is the sperm bank. I wondered if it had regular opening hours and what sort of conversations went on at the counter. "Oh, Mr Fee, can I have a quiet word, it's er, rather a delicate matter..... the account you see, there haven't been any deposits since it was opened..... Is there some sort of problem?". Then there was the rather mysterious process of banking a deposit, steady now. Discussions with younger members of the leukaemic clan hinted at the stark reality that was being locked in a room with a container and 'aids' (I'll leave that to your own warped imagination) to produce sufficient 'deposit' to keep the bank Manager happy! Hardly the ideal scenario for procreation and introducing a new soul into the world. Knowing what state I was in when initially diagnosed, I would have been struggling to produce anything even had the entire contents of my deepest fantasies been realised, which they weren't. My final ponderings were along the lines of how do you make a withdrawal? I decided that the double entendres were becoming too frequent so gave up at this point. Suffice to say, for the budding leukaemic it is an important point which can affect future plans and indeed individual lives for good. For individuals who crave the prospect of parenthood, the psychological impact on them must be massive.

Chapter Three

An Introduction to Hospital Life

The Ward

Ward 8, along with other wards dealing with haematological cancers at the Royal Victoria Infirmary (or RVI as it is known locally – there we go again on board the punchy abbreviation bandwagon) were living on borrowed time. Plans were afoot to move to the Freeman Hospital a few miles up the road to become a part of the Northern Centre for Cancer Care. This Centre of Excellence draws patients from a vast geographical area including Tyneside, Teeside, Northumberland, North and West Cumbria, North Yorkshire and there was even someone from North Lincolnshire.

The layout of the ward was based on the Victorian design, funnily enough, a long corridor ran for the majority of the length of the ward, off this lay treatment rooms and individual cubicles for female patients and those patients requiring isolation following bone marrow transplants. At the end of the ward was 'my patch'. Here the corridor gave way to a large open ward which was more like a sports hall. I preferred this setting due to the massive high ceiling and feeling of space, better than the modern claustrophobic design. Bed space by modern comparison was quite generous, the vast cavern area was, however noisier than its modern counterparts. There was a beautiful parquet floor which was polished daily by the amazing team of cleaning staff who did an incredible and most important job, minimising the risk of infection. No surface was left undusted, if you stood still you were likely to get polished.

My first visit to the ward saw me in my own cubicle which I thought to be quite acceptable, this, however, lasted one night only as it was needed by someone in greater need of it than I. So I was moved out into the open ward where I ended up in the bed next to the 'sluice'. For those uninitiated souls who have decided to read this out of a macabre fascination (a bit like those people who are frightened of snakes but still have to visit the reptile house at the zoo), the sluice is the room where the nursing staff dispose of the bedpans and commodes – that was the polite version, others were in use on the ward as I am sure you can imagine.

So, here I was, a hospital virgin, out on the open ward with six other inmates, some obviously veterans of a long hospital campaign and at ease with the routine in place. So, do I present with bluff or do I keep my head well and truly below the parapet and keep quiet. I opt for the latter and await developments. Those who want to talk soon do so, those who don't want to similarly make their feelings known. The game of eye contact tennis was quite fun, waiting for those who didn't want to speak to be having a crafty peek at what you were up to and getting them in full eye contact catching them unawares. The result was usually the recipient diving back behind the newspaper or other such diversory technique. I considered this a point gained, fifteen love etc. There would be occasions where a volley would take place, that was a brief look away followed by another peek, look away etc. Days were sometimes long and you had to take what entertainment there was in all its many guises.

I love different dialects. During my stays in Newcastle I became a 'hinnie'. This was a term used to address people as in "Are ye alreet hinnie?". I have previously been a 'love' in Yorkshire, a 'duck' in Nottingham and a 'marra' in West Cumbria and felt quite honoured to add a 'hinnie' to the list. The people of the North East have a genuine warmth about them, they do, however, tend to be quite loud, this appearing to be a widespread trait. I came up with the theory that maybe this was due to the previous heavy industries being so noisy that everyone had to shout to be heard. Either that or my hearing is just overly sensitive.

Football in the North East is the equivalent to a religion. The ward as I found out had both Newcastle and Sunderland fans in. Discussing football was found to be a no go area. I happened to be admitted the week of the Newcastle versus Sunderland match mentioning the score once and just managing to get away with it. There would not be a second time. Things started to get silly when a Leeds fan was admitted with a broken leg and was lucky to be discharged fairly soon with all remaining limbs intact.

There were pros and cons with having my treatment seventy miles away from home. The advantages included the fact that I was being treated in a Centre of Excellence and its associated resources, both human and otherwise. There is no doubt that these people whose care I was in were the best in their field. If I needed a scan I would be there as soon the porter collected me. I was given 5 star treatment. The main disadvantage was visiting. Friends and family had a long trek, those who made the effort were rewarded by an anaemic leukaemic with no hair but wearing a smile!!

Leukaemia is not discriminatory in who it attacks. There were businessmen on the ward who spent days sending global e-mails and an unemployed ex-nurse such as myself. A real microcosm of society existed on Ward 8. Some chose to speak others did not. Some formed friendships which were to last beyond the leukaemia, others found acquaintances on the ward a real help. Self help and support was found in the most unlikely places. Jim, a 6'4 bricklayer with some amazing tattoos introduced me to Life Mel honey, the worlds most expensive honey at nearly £40 for a small jar. Jim swore by it, "Boosts your immune system mate". How could I refuse?

Mary Poppins or Porridge ?

Ward 8 was lacking something though. A view ! For someone such as myself who likes being out in the great outdoors, a period of confinement such as this was made worse by the lack of a view. I love to watch scenes of life and all those little vignettes that watching such scenes offers. Here though, the only view was out onto Victorian rooftops. I half expected Mary Poppins to appear, or better still Dick Van Dyke perhaps trying to Americanise the Geordie accent having successfully murdered cockney.

There were days, of course when the mix of morphine and antibiotics meant that I didn't really give a hoot about any views as the majority of the day was spent in some other reality where Dick Van Dyke was a doctor and was using his sweeps brushes in a rather peculiar way as a remedy for constipation....Towards the end of my treatment it was sad that the ward began to have the feeling of a prison about it. My chemotherapy became the equivalent of doing porridge. I sussed out who 'Mr Mackay' was and there were several candidates for 'Fletch'. Instead of cigarettes there was a black market in wine gums. I would not survive a spell in prison !

The Dray Horse Society

This started as a joke on one of the wards I worked on during my psychiatric nursing career. My first day was met with "Whatever you do don't sit next to Harriet, she farts like a dray horse !" For the younger readers wondering what dray horses were, they were heavy horses that used to pull the carts delivering beer kegs to hostelries in the good old days of flat caps, woodbines and when the working class were allowed to do just that. So, on the ward on which I worked after this wisecrack, anyone with problems with flatulence joined Harriet in 'The Dray Horse Society'. Just as an aside, Harriet was a member of staff and was justifiably a founder member of the said society, and indeed was proud of her heritage in this respect.

As we live in litigious times I perhaps need to include a sort of disclaimer should any dray horses or their relatives be reading this and take hurt and deem such writings as slanderous and a general slur on their character. I thus unreservedly apologise should any heavy horses take offence at this and encourage them to take it in the light hearted way it was intended.

On Ward 8 the heady mix of hospital food, chemotherapy and antibiotics meant that The Dray Horse Society had a regular supply of honorary members. There were some, it has to be said, that were obviously long established members before they arrived. There was one member who arrived in the bed next to me in 'the wee small hours'. After a few days in the vicinity of this chap, I had visions of him attending The Dray Horse Society Annual Awards (the equivalent of the Oscars in the world of flatulence) and sweeping the board. I imagined him giving his acceptance speech, "I would like to thank my father for his support and for keeping this tradition alive....". The noise of that quivering sphincter letting forth with gusto I likened to being the equivalent to the lightning, the noxious aroma later reaching the nostrils the equivalent of the thunder. This constant sensory overload which included the snoring meant that there were many long nights. I began to time the gap between the sphinctoral volley and the inhalation of gases which would curl hair if I had some and surely could be used in some modern warfare scenario. The longest was 1 minute 15 seconds, the shortest 43 seconds......like I said it was a long night that.

Are Your Bowels OK ?

I am reminded of a scene whereby a husband is trying to surreptitiously purchase some exotic lingerie for his wife in a department store but cannot find the right size. Plucking up courage he asks the assistant if she has the size he is looking for. To his embarrassment the assistant holds up said lingerie and yells to her colleague at the other side of the department "The gentleman's after these in a size 12...". This gentleman was not me I hasten to add.

Back to Ward 8, the nurse undertaking her drug round parks her trolley in the middle of the ward. Due to the fact that I had required some laxatives the previous day ("Morphine bungs you up summat terrible" as a fellow inmate put it) I was thus treated with "Anything for your bowels John?". I was tempted to respond with "A bit louder nurse the chap at the far end of the corridor didn't quite catch it ". At least the larger group of visitors found it amusing. Welcome to the world of the hospital in-patient where nothing appears to be sacred. In case you're wondering yes I did and it worked.

Of Toilets and Showers

In the early days following diagnosis I was poorly. Pain was an ever present companion and tasks I usually did without batting the proverbial eyelid became mountains to climb. It never got totally dark on the ward but the morphine induced dream time meant that there was still the "Where on earth am I ?" scenario on waking. One minute I'm wandering around in an alternate reality dressed in cling film and floating somewhere approaching a blissful state (now I understand why people use drugs), the next minute the old family bladder problem means I'm back on the ward with a trek to the loo to undertake. I was definitely at the back of the queue when bladders were being handed out, mine appears to be the size of a walnut. Compare this with the major achievements in human history, Amundsen reaching the South Pole, Hillary reaching the summit of Everest, Neil Armstrong setting foot on the moon, such was the effort involved. I was in such a state, both physical and mental that a 20 yard walk (did I say walk) to the loo ranked amongst the greatest of human achievements, to aim and pass something once there would be the icing on the cake so to speak. Call me stubborn, full of male pride or just plain daft but some inner driver forbade me to succumb to using a bottle to pee into as someone would have to clear it away in the morning.

Let me guide you through such a pioneering moment in human history, my trek to the loo. Picture the scene then, drip stand attached to arm, T-shirt and boxer shorts in situ to preserve what modicum of dignity I had left. Phase one, the getting out of bed procedure. Still in somewhat of a drug induced haze and still flitting back to being dressed in cling film, I press the wrong button on the bed control panel and end up with my legs in mid air instead of my head. In the mayhem that ensued I drop the control panel and it clatters to the ground briefly bringing the dray horse next door out of his snorting and silence reigned briefly before he returned to galloping in some distant field. Not only do I now have my feet pointing to the ceiling but now I have lost my means of rectifying this. I lie there for a moment thinking about all those pioneers of human achievement that have gone before. I decided that accident proneness probably didn't go hand in hand with renowned adventurers. I decided that the Titanic would be more in my line, probably in some navigational capacity, maybe even as captain, "There are no icebergs here son…"

Given that the blood was by now flowing steadily to my brain and the cling film reality was fading (I'm sure that Freud would have written a whole series of books about me), my mental acuity returned and my male problem solving skills kicked in. At the bottom of the bed hooked onto the bed rail was a second bed control panel, one which the nursing staff could use to catapult you upward, downward or even seemingly re-create the old Corkscrew Rollercoaster ride of Alton Towers fame, depending on their like/dislike of the bed occupant. If I could unhook this with my feet I could rescue the whole situation. Trouble was my feet were now two feet in the air and subsequently above said rail and control panel. I mentally quivered at this point and began the slippery slope of negative thinking. I mused that it would be the equivalent of Amundsen thinking "What's the deal with this North Pole thing anyway?" and Hillary stating "We could always say the flag was blown off the top..." For me, this resulted in me nearly using the Nurse Call Buzzer which was handily placed to my left. I hang my head in shame as I write this but please recognise my human frailties. I snapped out of this dangerous thinking and gracefully swivelled myself to the sitting position using my good arm and my now very lean buttocks. It was a move reminiscent of Olga Korbut on the beam in those heady days of the 1972 Olympics. Phase one complete.

Phase two was to involve putting on slippers and disconnecting the drip stand and pump from the mains power supply, only I forgot that this was a necessity, driven from my mind by the fact that my slippers appeared to have walked to a position underneath my bed, this after having been left ever so neatly in a place ready for me to leap (I use the term lightly in this instance) into should some emergency arise. Quite what emergency never really was considered although on reflection, a small bladder, severe leg pain and the equivalent of a hike up Everest to empty said small bladder could be classed as an emergency should a directory of emergencies ever be compiled. I sat and pondered. If I got on the floor, such was my state that getting up would be like asking Edwina Currie to become Patron of The Egg Producers of GB, something that just wouldn't happen. So, barefoot it was then.

I stood, the room began to spin and the pain in my legs seemed to increase tenfold. I girded what loins I had left, gripped my old friend the drip stand and off we went taking our first faltering steps towards the summit....Unfortunately at this point the plug flew out of the pump on the drip stand immediately triggering the pump alarm. The dray horse awoke as did most of the ward. Despite only having three red blood cells in my body due to the anaemia I still managed to turn red. The human body really is amazing. By now though, the levels of adrenaline were surpassing that of morphine and I deftly stopped the alarm on the pump and proceeded on my way.

My walk, and I use the term lightly, has to be described in context. I was suffering severe leg pain at this time which increased on weight bearing and I could not straighten my legs fully so I looked like I was mid way though a version of 'The Funky Chicken' when on my way to the loo. To night nurse Lynne, though, my walking would have appeared to be the same as someone who had the misfortune to have been doubly incontinent. She paddled down the ward towards me, "Have we had an accident …." She whispered and then mouthed "…down below ?" I responded that this was my normal gait at present and then she was gone, a grey figure bearing her bedpan offering to the Temple of the Sluice….

The summit was in sight. It was then that I discovered that just when you think that life cannot get any worse, it can and does, with knobs on ! I had the only drip stand in the northern hemisphere with a squeaky sticking wheel and a tendency to go right instead of straight on. It may not seem much, but put into this context it is such straws that have left many a dromedary lying staring at the stars. Grown men have been seen to weep at such things. There were mutterings and much turning over in the beds around me. It was official, I was a Disturber of the Peace. Even the dray horse was giving me the evil eye amongst much huffing and puffing. Oh well, onward and upward as Hillary would have said. The summit at last, well a few feet away at least. The next problem was getting the drip stand into the cubicle as the disabled cubicle was in use. I somehow had to get me and my metal companion who was still wanting to go in the opposite direction into the toilet.

I headed into the cubicle first, so far so good, then pulled the drip stand which suddenly decided it would run smoothly resulting in its by now thoroughly cheesed off operator having the skin removed from his heels and very nearly doing a forward somersault down the toilet pan. So, the operation nearly complete, my summit experience was almost there, just the equivalent of the driving in of the flag on the highest peak on Earth to go then, yes the emptying of the walnut sized bladder which by now felt more like a football.

Chemotherapy can have strange effects on the process of passing urine – for those of a nervous and/or delicate disposition look away now please. All I will say in this instance was it was orange and also "it's frothy man" to recall some meaningless 1980's advert, the product of which I fail to recall and am not looking up but involved lager and a bear. When I say frothy I mean try having a pee after squirting a bottle of Fairy Washing Up Liquid down the loo and you will get the picture. I did joke to one of the nurses that if I had all the colours of my various chemotherapy at the same time (there was red, orange, green and blue), I could pee a rainbow. We were not amused however and went off tutting.

After all this excitement my body decided to withdraw what sparks of energy were left and so I was forced to sit down on the loo and contemplate the success of my achievement that night….there may be a book….a Booker Prize…..Morphine is wonderful stuff, I wondered if delusions of grandeur were a recognised side effect. So with heels chafed and sore, a now empty walnut sized bladder and a Booker Prize for best newcomer, I once again girded my rapidly diminishing loins and headed squeakily back to bed with my wandersome companion.

Of course, those of you following this somewhat surreal plot will be aware that there was still the small matter of the bed and its bizarre 'toes to ceiling' position I had left it in. I squeaked my way past the end of the bed and past my route to salvation in the form of a bed control panel hanging there cunningly disguised as a bed control panel. Reaching my bedside I sat in a wilted heap, energy spent and compared myself to those who on approaching the finishing line of the London Marathon suddenly look down and see strips of rubber where their legs had been and the 'Ministry of Funny Walks' begins much to everyone's amusement apart from themselves and their loved ones. Thus, here I was in a similar predicament, the race nearly over bar the final hurdle of getting into a bed where my legs would be two feet in the air. Getting the control panel was a bridge too far as it was behind my bedside chair and it would need some energy, a no go for me at this juncture.

Those of you from an engineering background would have fathomed out the solution several pages back. The solution, move the pillows to the feet end and sleep in reverse. That's what I did anyhow, much to the amusement of the night staff as they came round at 6am to take my observations, very nearly putting the blood pressure cuff on my leg and talking to my feet. It was a long night for all concerned. Back to Freud and the cling film, nurse the morphine please…

I struggled to shower every day during those early days of treatment due to me being so unwell and being hooked up to either chemotherapy or antibiotics or anti fungal drugs or…..the list seemed to be endless. When I did get there the showers themselves were something of an anathema. Just when you got lathered and ready for a rinse the shower would dry up. I worked out that whenever anyone in Newcastle ran a tap our showers died. The good news was that the itching had gone, disappeared, vanished, I could now have a hot shower, not, seemingly on Ward 8 though.

Institutionalisation – I was that Sheep

Generally speaking we all have some sort of routine in which we conduct our lives. Ward 8 was no exception to this in that it had a general timetable for meals, nursing interventions such as the regular taking of patient observations (that is temperature, blood pressure, pulse and blood oxygen levels) and consultant rounds. Within this regime there was a degree of flexibility, food could be brought in and consumed when wanted. In my case I resorted to squirrel like behaviour, hoarding biscuits and snack bars in my bedside cabinet, often consuming them under cover of darkness, merely because this was when I felt like eating and not through any nocturnal fetish type disorder. The first set of observations or 'obs' as they are known in the trade kicked off at 6am. Yes that was six in the morning. Lights out on a good day would be 11pm more often than not it would be 1am. They were long days.

It would appear that as soon as we enter a hospital ward the majority of us give away our power. There could almost be an exchange whereby as soon as the name band goes on, the recipient presents back a formal waiver of rights over their body. I am sure that if a nursing sister had wheeled a trolley onto the ward and announced that everyone were to receive an enema then pyjama bottoms would be round the ankles before the first rubber glove was donned. The other thing is why do we put our pyjamas on during the day when there is no need ? Answers on a postcard please. Studies have been carried out on the "Sick role" that many of us seem to adopt as soon as we cross the hospital threshold.

The more familiar I became with hospital life the more my power seemed to return. Lots of time to reflect led me to start to ask questions about what was happening to my body, what was being pumped into it, what did it do, why was it necessary and what delightful side effects could I expect ? I may have been classed as a nuisance but at the end of the day this was my body, the only one I have and I had the right to know what was happening. It was noticeable that further into their illness, some people found confidence to ask for copies of their blood results and to openly discuss and negotiate treatment plans. The Consultants did facilitate this where it was obvious that the individual patient wanted to know more and was taking an active and keen interest in their treatment. Others just rolled over with the "Do what you like Doc" type approach. No judgement, each to their own, we all cope in different ways.

The TV Remote

Channel surfing is a modern phenomena I am led to believe, usually a male specialism along with 'couch potatoism'. There is nothing quite like having the TV remote in hand, beer and snacks within easy reach and a multitude of channels to flick through- the domain of the modern male was complete. What a dilemma then, 7 males, one television and horror of horrors, only one remote control. There were, it has to be said, larger periods of time sometimes extending to days, when the television would remain inactive. This depended upon who was in and what day and time it was. Saturday nights for example used to see strategic planning from various parties to get in early for X-Factor and Match of The Day.

Strategies were inventive and diverse and in some cases obviously needed something akin to a criminal mind to draw up. One would entail grabbing the remote early on Saturday morning whilst everyone else was busy showering and dressing etc and storing said remote in one's bedside cabinet, furtively buried under a newspaper on a bedside table was a similar technique. "Anyone seen the remote ?" would be met with shakes of the head all round. MI5 would have had recruits aplenty on Ward 8. The most devious strategy observed was to remove the batteries from the remote rendering it inoperative. As the time of the programme the 'operative' wanted to watch approached, said operative suddenly found some batteries which they proceeded to slot into the remote, apparently donating them to the ward as if they were new and not the originals removed earlier. Such benevolence ! Just call me the ward mole…

The World of the Night Nurse

The culture and atmosphere of Ward 8 would change according to what was happening in terms of patients and staff on a particular shift. There would usually be a major change, often for the better with the introduction of ………..the night staff. Whether it was the lack of senior figure or merely the personalities involved it was difficult to say. However, a sense of fun was to prevail be it in the form of practical jokes, wisecracks and general all round good humoured banter. People responded, those who had presented as very unwell could be seen to rally merely by listening to the jocularity. The tasks were carried out efficiently and when emergencies arose these consummate professionals put on display the advanced skills and abilities which lurked behind the jovial facade and sense of fun.

Nights in hospital can be long and depressing affairs after lights out, particularly where pain and psychological discomfort are involved. The warmth shown by the nursing team at times when we are at our lowest ebb was deeply welcome. It was at times such as these that the fellow dressed in black dragging the scythe would appear and beckon me to follow him. I decided to stay, the night nurses helped me decide.

Chapter Four

Chemo!

Of Bone Marrow Biopsies

Those of a delicate constitution or those about to have a bone marrow biopsy either look away now or stick your fingers in your ears. The sample of bone marrow which is taken helps with diagnosis and, in between treatments it is used to check on the effectiveness of treatment i.e. is the patient 'in remission' where there is no sign of leukaemia and the bone marrow is working normally. I was fortunate in that I was in remission after each treatment session. The bone marrow sample is taken under local anaesthetic and is carried out by a doctor. Unfortunately for the poor patient, the bone and bone marrow cannot be anaesthetised. I quote from "Understanding Acute Myeloid Leukaemia" , a pamphlet produced by Cancerbackup, a registered charity and now part of Macmillan Cancer Support, which does invaluable work helping thousands of people with cancer in various ways. Here's what it says on the bone marrow sample/biopsy:

> *"You will be given a small injection to numb the area and the doctor will gently pass a needle through the skin into the bone. The doctor will draw a small sample of liquid marrow into a syringe. The doctor will then take a small core of marrow from the bone. It may be uncomfortable*

as the marrow is drawn into the syringe but this should only last a few seconds. You may feel bruised after the test and have an ache for a few days. This can be eased with mild painkillers."

My version, as you can probably imagine is slightly different. I had to lie on my left side with my knees drawn up, exposing my pelvic area. The 'small scratch' ploy used by the doctors to describe the local anaesthetic should be done under the Trades Description Act. One nurse described it to be nearer a bee sting which is probably more accurate. So, local anaesthetic applied (several small scratches later) and away we go with the heavy duty equipment. I didn't dare look at what was used but it felt and sounded like a corkscrew and a bicycle pump.

I have strong bones apparently, which is generally considered good but not to my advantage in this scenario with someone trying to bore through them. I was milk monitor at school in the days of free milk and used to get any bottles that were left. I was that calcium junkie. To get through my bone appeared to be the equivalent of drilling in exploration of oil, I half expected the doctor to be wearing a hard hat. So, the corkscrew employed successfully we were through, no bone marrow geyser in this instance though. The drawing up of bone marrow is difficult to describe. Very uncomfortable is the polite version, like a flock of starlings flying up the inside of your leg bone is another. One observant doctor commented "You're gripping the bed", enough said.

My first biopsy left me walking like an apprentice cowboy with bad piles for a week thereafter. The ones that followed weren't that bad. Some doctors were better than others it has to be said. A necessary evil to keep me here sums the process up nicely.

Cherryade, Lemonade or a Blue Wicked Sir?

The very word 'Chemo' strikes fear into those who have survived cancer, are suffering from this dreadful blight on mankind and probable terror into the hearts of those spared the disease, just about everybody then. So, "What is it really like then John" I hear you cry, curious about this modern terror which paradoxically saves lives. Grim, I would respond , very grim. More about that later, I shall leave you in suspenders.

For the leukaemic such as myself, the drugs I had were designed to basically kill off my bone marrow as mine had decided to go pear shaped by producing cancerous cells. So, these drugs killed off my red and white cells leaving me highly anaemic with no immune system whatsoever. Hence I had to have numerous transfusions of blood and platelets and live like a hermit to avoid infections.

I won't bore you with the names of all the cytotoxic drugs which were pumped into me over those months. Some took an hour or two to get into my system, others took 12 hours. My worst treatment involved five days of constant chemotherapy, 24 hours a day, time out for showers had to be negotiated with nurses. The colours of the drugs were interesting to say the least. Some were clear (lemonade), red (cherryade), green (creme de menthe), blue (blue wicked) and orange (orangeade, naturally). Psychologically, naming them as such appeared to lessen the fear factor and took away the fact that I was being slowly poisoned to the point of death. I reiterate what has already been said within this book and by others, make no bones about it, chemotherapy is brutal and grim.

Observing others on the ward, as we humans are prone to do, purely in an attempt to gain an insight into how others coped I was left none the wiser. Withdrawal from the world seemed to be one way as in the head under the covers ploy, hoping it was all a nightmare and on emerging from the duvet it would turn out to have been all a bad dream. Everyone seemed to struggle at some point despite initial bravado and a stiff upper lip which invariably would quiver at some point during treatment. For me the focus was on when this treatment session would finish and I would be free again.... For leukaemia, chemotherapy goes deep, after all you can't get much deeper than bone marrow !

Name Rank and Serial Number

It would start from somewhere up the corridor, like the beginnings of an earth tremor, life on the ward would stop for an instant as the sound of the wheels over the parquet floor resembled a train rumbling over the tracks gradually got louder. The noise grew up to a crescendo until.....the Chemo Trolley burst out onto the open ward. It's attendants, always in yellow aprons, always in two's, medical notes under the arm, eyes searching to see what state their next victim was in. All eyes would in return be focused on the trolley and its operators, either surreptitiously from behind a book, newspaper or similar cover or quite openly for those either in the early stages of treatment in the "This is a piece of cake, I'm hard" mindset or gripped with such fear that they just can't help themselves but look (similar to watching Dr Who from behind the settee).

Whoever came, there was the collective sigh of relief accompanied by rustling of newspapers, visits to the loo or striking up of conversations from the lucky ones who had escaped the horror of the trolley on that occasion. Then the ritual would begin. "Name rank and serial number" was the regular request from the nurses to make sure they were poisoning the right victim. It probably started off as a chortle, a guffaw, an ice breaker in what must be a difficult situation for the nurses presented with an inwardly frightened/terrified person despite whatever variety of fronts were on display. After four or five months what chink of humour that had existed in the early days had long since gone on the same train as the 'This hospital food ain't bad' and 'These beds are quite comfy' delusions. The fact that there is a check is comforting in that it gives you confidence that you are getting the right poison.

At this point I need to perhaps explain my reasoning for using the term 'poison' whilst referring to the chemotherapy. That is how I saw it from day one and still see it to this day. Make no bones about it, I am deeply grateful the said poison was available for me along with the knowledge, skills and experience of the medical team with whom I came into contact. I have a future thanks to them. Despite all the vast knowledge of medical science, treatments involving chemotherapy are brutal, and, ultimately people suffer. Perhaps I show a degree of resentment which comes across, that is because I know that there are other treatment modalities which can support the body through this regime and perhaps make it more bearable and ease the suffering for people.

The Phantom of The Opera – A Nursing Parody

If I suffered any type of heart defect it would have manifested on this particular day. Early in my treatment I was receiving chemotherapy along with a cocktail of antibiotics due to various infections. These drugs along with the morphine and antihistamine meant that lucid and coherent were becoming distant cousins who have moved out to stay with a distant aunt in the country for a while. I came out of my drug induced haze to find two nurses peering at me, one wearing a full face clear mask. "Does the bed need some welding" I slur, due to the intoxicating drug cocktail and having my tongue decide to glue itself to the roof of my mouth. "We're being audited so we have to go through the proper procedure". The subsequent conversation   (somewhat one sided due to said tongue rebellion) establishes that the full face mask was to prevent eye damage in the event of the chemo bag rupturing and splashing. What was this stuff being pumped into me ? What about my eyes ? I returned to my antibiotic haze dreaming of nurses in space suits with syringes the size of cricket bats........Freud would be booking the next 10 sessions at this point !

Lethargic Lenny & The Frozen Arm

"This isn't so bad". My initial thoughts as the first bag of chemotherapy entered my body through a canula in my right arm. I was lulled into a false sense of security as two hours later I turned into "Lethargic Lenny". The tiredness associated with chemotherapy is not the sort of 'end of a busy day sit down with a glass of wine to watch the TV feeling tired' type scenario. This is heavy duty tiredness, fatigue, lethargy man! Walking to and from the toilet, a trip of about 25 metres, used up my resources for a few hours. What energy you do have is quickly used up, getting in and out of bed then becomes the equivalent of a novice runner with no training being on the start line of the London Marathon. So Lenny became a regular part of my psyche. A few months post treatment he is still a daily reminder of how serious an illness it is. For someone who was physically very active I would argue that it is even harder to accept that my 'get up and go' has done just that. I became a couch potato in a matter of hours.

At first, I have to admit that couch potatoism was quite an acceptable way of being. Being diagnosed with Leukaemia in one sense gave me a legitimate reason for taking time out to rest. No one would expect me to be doing a great deal, I could rest with reason and accept the waves of sympathy that initially flowed. Having always found it difficult to truly relax, here I was being forced to take time out. Enjoyable as it initially was this would turn into frustration later in the treatment cycle especially when we would enjoy our best spring weather wise in years. There are positives, as always, the main one being time to write this book, which by now you are hopefully grateful I did.

Having been admitted to hospital on the Thursday in a whirlwind of emotions and hormones, I began chemotherapy on the Saturday, the first day it was available from the hospital pharmacy. I was booked in to have a Hickman Line® inserted into my chest the following Wednesday. This is a surgical procedure which has to be done under X-Ray machine to ensure it has been correctly fitted. The line serves as a means to give drugs more directly into the bloodstream as it enters a major vein just above the heart. In the meantime then, the chemotherapy was given through a canula on the back of my right hand. It was during this time that the chemotherapy damaged my right arm. I recall it being painful at the time it was going through and into my arm but it was not until afterwards that my arm swelled and I was unable to bend it properly without excruciating pain. A thrombosed vein was diagnosed with phlebitis.

It was the pain associated with this that led me onto the painkiller trail. Past experience of painkilling medication was that doctors normally started off with very mild painkillers and worked their way up in potency until one they found one that worked. Here it was clearly acceptable to go straight for the hard stuff, hence my introduction to the world of opiates. The pain used to be worse at night and so I would use the nurse call system to request some pain relief. The vision in uniform would appear as an angel bearing a route to heaven. It is good stuff! It would give me pain relief and also wonderful feeling of euphoria. Nothing mattered when this stuff was coursing about my system, even the dray horses' noxious gases took on the aroma of rose petals. It was very good stuff this !

So I became a drug user. I was on a slippery slope! There was a great temptation when the pain had eased to carry on with the morphine. No I didn't is the answer to your question. Like all drugs, though, there are side effects. In my case it 'bunged me up' so to speak, after not opening my bowels for four days things were getting desperate, despite several visits to the loo where I could have read War and Peace twice over. It also affected my bladder, giving me the urge to pass water but nothing happened until I returned to my bed when the urge returned with that "accident is looming" type feeling. For my visitors, it was to prove interesting in that they encountered a euphoric leukaemic with eyes on stalks one minute who turned into a snoring heap the next. Interesting times……

The Hickman Line® Experience

"Hello I'm Dr Blah Blah". I was lying on a trolley with one of those gowns designed by hospital gurus to highlight the fact that what dignity you once had was left at the door on admission. You know the ones, they tie up at the back but leave your bum on parade for all to see. Whether it was the morphine/antibiotic haze or merely my rebellious streak was difficult to tell but I had my gown on so it was tied at the front. My thinking was that as they were about to stick a tube in my chest, I could open the gown and away they would go. Logic appears to get lost in larger institutions I have found.

The figure bending over me wore full theatre dress, that is the gowns, hat and nice shiny white Wellingtons as modelled on ER, Casualty or Holby City, take your pick. Whichever you chose they must be designed to fill the incumbent on the trolley with abject terror. It certainly worked in my case. This little scenario was constructed so as to inform me on what was about to happen and to get me to sign my life away in the form of the Consent to Treatment documentation.

I quote from the Cancerbackup pamphlet again to explain about the line I was to have inserted into my chest.

> "To make it easier to give the chemotherapy drugs, and to avoid having to have frequent injections, a plastic tube (called a Central or Hickman® Line) can be put into a vein in the chest. The line is put in under a general or local anaesthetic and, apart from a stiff shoulder, which you may have for a couple of days, should be completely painless. Once it is in place, the central line is either stitched or taped to your chest to prevent it from being pulled out of the vein. Drugs are given through the tube directly into your bloodstream. The line can stay in place for many months.....
> Blood can be taken from the line for testing and blood transfusions can be given through it."

Sounds straightforward doesn't it, and, for the majority of leukaemics it is, apparently. Are you getting the feeling that mine is a slightly different version, well you guessed correctly. The doctor who was to carry out the procedure ran through the process like a well oiled used car salesman, designed to leave you brimming with confidence that the gowned apparition peering over the trolley had obviously done thousands of these before without problem. Having signed my consent to treatment form, I was left for twenty minutes while everything was prepared. Out in the corridor where the acoustics amplified the noises issuing from the theatre, my brain interpreted the sounds reaching it with unreassuringly vivid pictures of machetes and bow saws being gathered together in readiness.

Eventually I was wheeled in by the nurse who was there to monitor my pulse, blood pressure and blood oxygen levels at intervals throughout the procedure. I also was relying on this nursing type person to give me some sort of psychological reassurance throughout…. "Your gowns on the wrong way round". I was immediately transported back to my junior school playground and a certain Mrs Jackson who used to strike the fear of God in me even though I was innocent , although I'm sure that breathing was a sin in her book. "Well its got to come off anyway" and said gown was duly removed, a blanket was used to preserve what modicum of dignity I had left. I mused on the fact that the gown could have been undone and moved to expose my chest, but then decided that this was clearly a case of 'We've been doing it this way since the hunter gatherer days when knuckles were for dragging along the cave floor and we're not going to change now….'. I made a mental note to check the sign on the door of the theatre on the way out to check this was not the psychiatric wing for delusional patients with obsessive tendencies, but that would have needed a long sign.

The doctor in whose hands my comfort lay, both physical and equally important psychological comfort, appeared complete with mask and colleague whom she began to instruct in the gentle art of central line insertion. The old 'small scratch' ploy was used again for the local anaesthetic and then she proceeded to jab as though this was the world darts championship final. "I think that's one hundred and eighty" I quipped, trying to bring some frivolity into the situation. The silence that followed conjured up the scene of a deserted wild west town with tumbleweed blowing down the main street, a distant bell rings....... Guess that humour was a no go area here. I mused again and decided that musing was a hidden art at which I was beginning to excel. I had suddenly become a non person, a lump of body, an inanimate object there to be jabbed, cut, prodded and so on before a plastic tube is inserted. The doctor jabbered on to her colleague about sterile procedures, "A small cut here ....and this is where we start the tunnelling". Nobody had mentioned or even hinted at 'tunnelling' up until now and I voiced my concerns to that effect. "Tunnelling", I was patronisingly told as if a three year old is familiar with such run of the mill things, "is what we call the pushing of the line through the muscle which eventually grows around it and holds it in place". From this point on I decided I was an obvious inconvenience, the only conversation came in the form of the nurse at my side....."Cuff on your arm inflating" every five minutes, some psychological reassurance huh!

The procedure grew physical as I was pummelled and pushed and again mused what life must be like at the bottom of a rugby scrum. What faith I had in this gowned introvert disappeared when she exclaimed "Do you remember we had one like this last week ?", and turning to the recipient of her knowledge and expertise further stated "We get a really tough one about once a month, I'll have another go" and life at the bottom of the scrum returned. Their conversation turned to a certain Alison, who, apparently was good in such situations. It was concluded that Alison should be sent for. "Yes, let's have Alison here" I piped up. Said Alison duly arrived and retrieved the whole situation. Stitches were inserted and I was duly wheeled outside into the corridor to practise my newly acquired hobby of musing, feeling like I had experienced an encounter with the All Blacks.

Some five minutes later the nurse appeared. "We just want to check everything was OK for you? Was there anything we could have done differently?" – a sort of customer service process! I followed the national stereotypical Brit, "No, no it was fine thanks." Some complaint eh!

Of Platelets and Transfusions

"Hello Mr Fee", the voice belonged to a figure which had materialised at the foot of the bed and I awoke with a start. He drew the curtains around the bed as though this prevented anyone from hearing. "I'm Dr Blah Blah" strange name I thought , maybe he's related to Hickman line woman as I started to rouse from my morphine/antibiotic/infected haze. "We've looked at your platelets" he continued, that's nice I thought. They're at 4 !" he exclaimed. "Do I get a gold star then or is that figure behind you with a black cloak and a scythe something to be concerned about ?". "Normal levels" he went on "Are in the range of 140 upwards, yours are 4 !" he exclaimed again perhaps thinking I had missed the gravity of the situation first time round. "We'll get some ordered for you as soon as, ok, toodle pip" and with that the ghost like figure and his accomplice with the scythe toddled off.

Platelets are very small non-nucleated discs which contain a variety of substances that promote blood clotting which causes haemostatis (cessation of bleeding). Are you impressed with my medical prowess ? It's amazing what you can learn about your own body in such circumstances. The human body is truly amazing. So, the reason my legs looked like I'd been beaten with a wire brush, that my nose was full of semi-congealed blood (sorry for those with a delicate constitution) and my gums were bleeding was down to me only having a few of my platelet friends circulating. Those left were fire fighting and were probably about to strike due to increased workload and working hours with no increase in remuneration. Basically, I was bleeding to death. The first bag of straw coloured liquid, the platelets, arrived and were transfused into me. A platelet has a hard life and a short life, lasting only on average between 8 to 11 days, hence the need for constant monitoring and transfusions over the coming days, weeks and months.

I awoke in a daze with my head against the toilet door, I had gone for a pee and then felt violently nauseous and began to sweat profusely so that my T-shirt was ringing wet. I decided that whatever was about to happen (including meeting my maker) would be better done from a sedentary position. I had passed out and must have looked like Captain Mainwaring in Dad's Army, the scenes where he appears from a crowd with his glasses askew looking somewhat dishevelled. I pulled the red cord hanging before me and got a wheelchair ride back to my bed.

Anaemia goes with the territory for the leukaemic. I could have auditioned for "Night of the Living Dead" due to my ghostly pallor. The tiredness and breathlessness are constant companions for the anaemic leukaemic. Haemaglobin (Hb) is a complex protein-iron compound found in the blood which carries oxygen to the cells from the lungs and removes carbon dioxide from cells to the lungs. Generally, normal range of haemoglobin is between 13 and 18, there are variances between men and women. My levels were 7.5 when I passed out ! I came to realise that I got increasingly breathless even when not moving when my levels dropped below 10. Below 8 or 9 for me was getting into dangerous passing out parade type territory. Without the generosity and self sacrifice of blood donors I would not be here now. Thank you ! I was that vampire.

The Foetal Position, A Rusty Mouth & Floaters

Go around any hospital ward throughout the country and I guarantee you will find at least one person lying in the foetal position. At some level, when we are suffering we seem to return to this shape to gain some modicum of comfort in our hour of need. Ward 8 was no exception, indeed probably 8 out of 10 inmates would exhibit this position on a daily basis, myself included. Maybe it is the psychological equivalent of withdrawal, physically trying to make oneself as small as possible. No doubt some boffin has devoted his or her life to such matters and has ended up wondering why nobody sits next to them at parties.

With leukaemia, the chemotherapy treatment is designed to destroy your bone marrow in various degrees depending on the treatment regimen being employed. It affects everyone differently, my own experience was to become Lethargic Lenny but also to have aches throughout my muscoskeletal system. For those of you who have suffered from full blown influenza (as opposed to the man flu variety), the sort which puts you in bed for a fortnight, that is like the aching I experienced. This is what led me to curl up like a ball.

If you were to ask me what were the worst elements of my cancer journey, it is difficult to answer. For me it was the accumulation of all the symptoms of the leukaemia and all the side effects of the chemotherapy which added up to produce a miserable little bunny. I don't know about you but one of my great pleasures in life is a good nosh. A nice meal is, for me, one thing I can look forward to and thoroughly enjoy. To take away your taste is thus to take one of the pleasures of life. There is a famous Scottish soft drink "made in Scotland from girders". Have you ever sucked on a rusty nail – welcome to my world!

The cravings for cheeseburgers and Cumberland sausage baguettes which were realised when I returned home were such a huge disappointment as everything tasted as though it had been seasoned with rust, such was the effect of chemotherapy. The whole eating experience from smelling the food cooking, getting those gastric juices running, the anticipation of the meal on its way was all shattered by the first bite into the iron steak. I became convinced there was an underground butchers society specialising in chemotherapy meat. "What today sir, we have rusty sirloin, maybe some filing sausage or we've just got some cast iron flavoured burgers for the more discerning palate" ..... Things were getting serious when food merely became something to force down to keep me alive with no modicum of pleasure. I became 'Disappointed of Cumbria'.

Serious illness can affect many parts of the body. Before I was diagnosed I became aware of dots before my eyes. I had always had one little spot on my eye which I remember having as a child and used to play games trying to look at it which ended up with frustration as when your eye moves to try and focus on it, the spot moves, always avoiding a direct look. We made our own fun back then!! So my long standing dot was joined by no less than six companions. I guess my original solitary dot would need some type of therapy to help it integrate into what was becoming a small community. It must be difficult having been a loner all these years to suddenly have to socialise .....

Floaters are spots that appear to drift in front of the eye and are caused by a shadow cast onto the retina by debris. The sudden onset of several floaters is often indicative of serious disease. Their technical name is 'Muscal Volitantes'. Impressed? So, here I was with my original floater being joined by a number of friends, assuming that they all get on. A few months later I would be diagnosed with a fairly serious illness! To play my advanced version of "Chase the Floater 4", I needed a plain background - blue skies are perfect, as was the magnolia ceiling on Ward 8. It's amazing what you can do to stave off boredom .... I am now getting out more you will be pleased to know.

I Was that Mushroom .... A Fungal Attack

I had always felt like a mushroom 'fed on bull**** and kept in the dark'. That this manifested on my physical being was probably appropriate. It all began in the early 1980's when my thumbnail on my left hand and then my toe nails were attacked with a fungal infection. For those who like detail and to impress friends with such, its technical name is Onychomysis, a fungal infection of the nails. This would be painful at times, particularly in Winter as the nail bed would often split, ouch! My feet were not spared and the skin on them became brittle and would split, often on the heel in Winter. Finally, it would flare up around my groin, 'down below', in hot weather. I learnt to live with it, cream would help with my 'down below' outbreaks when they flared up. Back then the remedies suggested for my nails by my GP all failed.

I went to see a Naturopath in February 2008 due to the itching I was experiencing. I was riddled with Candida Albicans. This is a yeast like, microscopic fungal organism normally present in the mucous membranes of the mouth, the intestinal tract and the skin of healthy people. This is what leads to ladies suffering problems 'down below' with vaginal thrush. I was put on a strict diet free from yeast and fungi and sugar. This along with a natural antifungal agent rid me of my mushroom status and gave me my nails back. Whether the itching was linked to this is difficult to tell but it did grow less.

Part of the routine treatment for the leukaemia was to give anti viral and anti fungal drugs. Our immune system would normally tackle any invasion such as these, when that goes you could be in trouble. At the time of diagnosis my immune system was severely compromised, in fact it had probably resigned due to excessive work load in the form of infections such as folliculitis and oral thrush – the fungal attack had re-commenced. I had also developed a lump on my neck which grew on a daily basis. Various scans proved inconclusive and various antibiotics failed to tackle my growing problem which was becoming painful and helped me embark on the morphine road to Euphoriaville. Eventually I was trialled on an intravenous antifungal drug which did the trick. Apparently this was very expensive, I was drawing on my National Insurance big time!

I have definitely been a hobbit in a previous life as I love mushrooms. Unfortunately I have chosen to give them up due to my predisposition to become one! The plus side? I have nice nails on my hands and feet and lovely soft feet, and no itching. I am now out in the light and avoid bull**** at all costs!

Testing Times

As mentioned previously, the care I received was second to none. If any investigations were needed I was there quicker than you could say 'hop into the wheelchair please Mr Fee'. There were x-rays, ultrasound scans and a CT scan. In some surreal kind of way, these escapades meant a trip out, a different view, a chat with the porter (if they were up to communication and if I felt well enough to converse) and something out of the ordinary hum drum existence of ward life.

Porters came in all shapes, sizes and ages and with very different styles of customer service. Take Bob, for example, he gave me a running commentary from leaving the ward to arriving at x-ray. He was more like a museum tour guide the amount of history and related information given freely without prompting. I was waiting for him to launch into the French and German versions but Geordie was all I got. Unfortunately, I had no loose change to tip him. Bob was a therapy in his own right and made me feel better by taking my focus off where I was going and more importantly, where I had just left.

Keith and Trevor were very different fellows. Keith did not speak – whether he could or not I never actually established. The vocal chords could form some noise in the form of a grunt, but from day one it was obvious that communication skills was not on the interviewing panels list of either essential or desirable attributes when Keith was taken on. I gave up trying. Trevor was the archetypal hard done by British worker, a role he obviously was destined for at an early stage. If you were thinking that leukaemia was a serious life threatening problem you would be sadly mistaken. Ten minutes in the company of said Trevor the Porter – "Did I tell you I've five kids, it's hard you know" …. - had you feeling as if you had a slight sniffle compared to his tales of woe. Maybe he was a psychologist in disguise. Certainly he would not go down well at a comedy club. I was losing the will to live …….

The Royal Victoria Infirmary is just like it says on the tin, a Victorian hospital. The corridors are long and in mid-winter would be suitable for penguins and polar bears. So, whenever I was to go for any test I would be wrapped up in blankets not unlike some disaster victim you see on a news report huddled in the background. On occasions when I had passed out I would be given a sick bowl to take with me, although I never actually used it I probably would have filled said bowl ten times over! Perhaps it was some sort of status symbol, it certainly got us a lift to ourselves, unfortunately I was with Trevor the Porter, luckily it didn't get stuck!

X-ray staff are like any others, some good, some not so. It was a bit like a production line. My condition and the fact that I looked like I had hours to go before persuading St Peter that my name was in his book somewhere, perhaps under the 'tried hard but was easily misled' section, meant that what queues were there were crashed quite rapidly. Chest x-rays involved standing up, a feat in itself on occasions, and slamming your chest against a freezing plate whilst the technician unreassuringly disappears into a cubicle in the far corner of the room before pressing the button. I suppose seeing a ghostly apparition covered with blankets and sporting the latest design in cardboard sick bowl was a bit different from the usual fractured this or that.

My growing neck had the doctors puzzled and me looking like I was constantly turning right with head cocked to one side. It was decided I would go for an ultrasound. It was a Saturday, hence the ultrasound department was effectively shut except for emergencies like me. I've never been an emergency before, this was uncharted territory for a boy from the backwoods ….. Porter and I arrived down a darkened corridor. A door opened and a head popped out, "This way please". Porter deposited my notes with the body to which the head was attached, a lovely lady doctor who got me to lie on the bed and proceeded to scan my neck, after applying gel and then using the hand held scanner against my bulging neck. The pain was excruciating, I confess that I cried. The results remained inconclusive, nothing nasty was present though which was a relief. I waited for a while before Bob the porter and a much more pleasant journey through the arctic tunnels ensued.

One side effect of chemotherapy is damage to the heart, some side effect eh! As I was passing out more than the doctors would have liked, if there is such an acceptable level, I was to go for an ultrasound scan of my heart. This came about after passing out in the chair next to my bed. It was the day after my birthday and Sandra had stayed overnight with our good friends Denise and John who live in Ashington, within the locality. She had returned earlier than usual that morning and was able to witness my dying swan escapade, alerting staff. I came around with the ward sister Jill, two inches from my nose shouting me. I don't know who was more surprised when I came around, myself or Jill. I was jokingly told that as I had received so much attention the previous day, that of my birthday, this was no way to behave to gain attention ! So, I was sent immediately for an ultrasound scan of my heart and, yes folks, I do have one, a very nice example if I may be so bold.

My neck continued to cause bewilderment amongst the medical team. It was prodded and poked and I was subsequently brought down from the ceiling with the promise of morphine. It was not a pleasant time. X-ray, ultrasound, next came the CT scan of my neck and upper torso (it stands for Computerised Tomography, for those who have to know such things and are good at pub quizzes). I was trussed up in the usual fashion and off we went, the grunting Keith and me off to the CT scanner, 3 miles from Ward 8. I threw some bread at the penguins and we eventually arrived in a corridor with a queue of equally ill looking people. Keith grunted to those behind the desk which appeared to mean something, threw my notes into my lap and off he trundled to his next in-depth conversation. Even though I felt rough, there were people here with drips, oxygen masks, in beds, virtually unconscious. I was no longer an emergency in such company and would have to wait.

People around me were given drinks of fluid containing a dye to enhance the imagery of the scan. When my turn came, about an hour or so later, and feeling generally awful, I was told that the dye would be given to me through my Hickman Line®. At least this thing in my chest was coming in handy. I lay on the treatment table and had a line attached to my line ready for the dye to go in. "It will feel a bit uncomfortable" one of the operators said. Call me paranoid if you like, but when people said things like this to me it usually meant a rough ride.

The CT scanner is a circular doughnut like structure through which the victim passes on a table, full of dye to highlight whatever part of your anatomy was to be scanned, for me that meant neck and upper torso. The "It will be a bit uncomfortable" was a twenty second burning sensation throughout my body followed by a severe headache. Again, as with x-rays, everyone disappeared out of the room and I was left to muse, at which

I was approaching PhD level. Dr of Musology sounded quite good. The scan showed I was generally ok, although I couldn't say I felt it at the time. So, I was prodded, poked, photographed and scanned, all to help me along the road to recovery. Such service was exemplary.

Slimmers World

It is widely acknowledged that chemotherapy affects most peoples appetite, I was one of those people who joined the involuntary slimming world of the cancer sufferer. I had already begun to lose weight before diagnosis, as those astute readers will know, having suffered with acute oral thrush which left my mouth so painful I was unable to eat properly. It was here that my crash diet really got underway, quite successfully it has to be said.

My first taste of hospital food either lulled me into a false sense of security or I was completely delusional in my thinking. Probably the latter, on reflection. My mouth was recovering somewhat at this stage and I had a salad that first evening which didn't seem too bad. Being a semi-vegetarian in that I still eat fish, the daily menu appeared to cater quite well for me. Breakfast on the ward included a full cooked breakfast if desired, dinner and tea varied from sandwiches to full cooked meals. Those first few days I was telling everyone that the food was ok, I was eating better than I had been. Then, chemotherapy happened!

For me, chemotherapy left me feeling nauseous yes, but worse in some respects was the way it affected my appetite.

Basically it left in a matter of hours. I was introduced to the concept of TAS, that is Trolley Avoidance Syndrome and refers to the inability to tolerate hot food and the subsequent need to avoid the smell emanating from the meal trolleys, which would leave me feeling pretty ghastly. I soon gave up ordering meals although a tray would still be sent up, something to do with pre-historic planning systems apparently. Coping strategies included timing a trip to the toilet with the arrival of the trolley, this would often result in being tracked by a member of staff whilst on the loo to ascertain whether I wanted anything to eat. In the words of Jim Royle of the Royle family series, "Can't I even have a **** in peace?"

My eating habits changed depending on which chemotherapy regime I was on. For the first few weeks, I felt better at night and so became a 'nocturnal nosher'. At that time I craved flavoured crisps, sweet cereal bars and plain biscuits. These would be consumed under cover of darkness, somewhat furtively to avoid disturbing other inmates. The acoustics in the ward meant that a bite on a crisp at 3am reverberated like thunder. I had to use the 'under the duvet' system. I gathered a squirrels pantry of goodies in my drawers, so much so I had no room for clothes.

The problem was that my tastes changed. I started having severe cravings for meat, particularly burgers and sausages. Someone in the next bed had a cheeseburger brought in. My pacifist beliefs went up in a smoke, I could have killed! Maybe it was my body telling me I needed meat and protein in particular. I learnt quickly that mornings weren't too bad and so had beans on toast for breakfast, this would be all I would eat on most days until the munchies set in during the hours of darkness.

At my worst I lost 1½ stone, not much in comparison to some people. The advice of the dieticians was to cram the calories. Here was I being given permission to eat cream cakes, chocolate, high fat foodstuffs and I couldn't manage them!! Life can be cruel at times. There is a book entitled *"Healthy Eating During Chemotherapy"*. It is by food writer Jose van Mil and Christine Archer-Mackenzie, a research psychologist and radiologist, both of whom have cared for husbands with cancer. This book is based on personal experience and has more than 100 simple, appealing recipes. After chemotherapy my immune system would gradually fade to zero, a slightly disturbing time during which I had to avoid certain foodstuffs such as blue cheeses, probiotic yoghurts, raw unpeeled fruit and vegetables and much, much more. Life got complicated! At least the local butcher accepted our custom after we had deserted him some 4 years ago.

On commencing chemotherapy I was encouraged to drink at least 3 litres of fluid per day. The hospital water was basically filtered tap water and soon grew warm in the ward environment. Its taste was pretty disgusting and seemed to get worse the warmer it got. It was at this stage that I entered the world of the Lucozade™ junkie. I was able to keep a store of soft drinks in the ward fridge and would often have a trip down the corridor returning with my bounty. Deep within me I think that the underlying reason for me to drink so much was an attempt to flush this poison out of my system.

"Flush Me Off Please Nurse"!

Being attached to a drip is a challenging experience. You will already be familiar with the expedition of going to the loo attached to said drip and the accompanying stand. I could not work out whether all the stands had dodgy wheels and a tendency to turn left or right or whether it was just my luck to keep getting a bad one. Certainly other inmates made it look easy, a bit like top sportspeople at the top of the game and the way they inspire misguided aspirants under the 'crikey that looks easy, must have a go' scenario. One of the aims of the leukaemic receiving chemotherapy, then, is to get rid of this five wheeled buddy as soon as. That's where we hit a small problem ...... the nurse's workload and the system for getting the thing disconnected.

It would have been nice to have been able to disconnect the drip from your own Hickman Line® once it had finished. Unfortunately it needed a nurse to disconnect the tube and then flush your Hickman Line® with a saline solution. This had to be done under sterile conditions, hence a trolley had to be set up in preparation and it had to fit in with their current workload. The chemo would run through a pump which would signal its finish by sounding an alarm. Some had slightly different tones, on one occasion there were about five pump alarms sounding, it sounded rather like the William Tell Overture. A woman who sneezed sounding like a neighing horse had the scenario complete.

The pump alarm would get switched off by whichever member of staff happened to be in the area. Then came .... The Wait.

There was a whiteboard in the nurse's clinical room, those requiring chemo and those requiring 'a flush' went on there also. Allegations that chocolate exchanged hands for moving up the list are outrageous and I utterly refute any suggestions of foul play, twas merely a slip of the dry wipe marker, obviously. At the end of the day it was often down to the personalities of the nurses on duty. A few could be won over by a whimpering pathetic individual pleading for a shower. (I played this role rather well, it received critical acclaim on the ward). Others dismissed the strategy and probably demoted the budding Olivier down the flushing off league for being so audacious.

Believe it or not this was one of my main stressors during my inpatient days. If I thought someone else had jumped the queue I would trundle off to the loo muttering about the unfairness of life etc. Some of my chemo was run over long periods, up to 22 hours for example. Delays in getting started, as the chemo had to be ordered and mixed by the pharmacy on a few occasions, meant I had to spend extra days in hospital. Welcome Mr Grumpy of Grumpsville! I had to reflect that it wasn't as if the nurses were sitting down having tea or coffee all day, they were lucky to get breaks some days. The problem was me adjusting to life in an institution. Value what freedom you have in your life!

Hair Today, Gone Tommorrow!

Ask anyone for a side effect of chemotherapy and I guarantee that 'loss of hair' would be the response. It's a fact, from day one of the chemotherapy treatment I was informed of all the side effects, hair loss being included. More bearable for men than women I would suggest. So when I started bunging up the plughole in the shower with hair, I knew something was amiss. My pillow took on the appearance of some strange grey haired animal. Yes, it was beginning to come out, in clumps! I took up the nurse's offer of shaving my hair off, better, I thought, to do it under my terms than to wait until my head looked like a patchwork quilt. So, off we went, nurse with clippers duly shaved my head. There wasn't much point in the nurse doing the usual 'is that alright sir' routine with a mirror for obvious reasons, but I was intrigued.

I casually sauntered to the toilets to see what damage the clippers had caused. Wearing my hair short anyway, I mused that it wouldn't look that much different. Oh my God! All I needed was an orange robe and I would be looking at a Tibetan monk. On second thoughts, with the wing nut ears there was a definite look of Yoda out of the Star Wars™ films. At least I would be alright for any fancy dress parties over Christmas. It was a psychological blow, joking apart, I feel for women who lose their hair, at least there are enough men out there with a challenging hairline for me not to stand out too much. It was no joke in mid-winter having no hair so I took to wearing a variety of head gear. I am not a hat sort of person so therefore I was introduced into the world of ridicule.

A shaved head and a corpse like pallor does tend to get you noticed when you are out and about though. The lack of eyebrows and eyelashes really makes you stand out. It would become an amusing exercise to catch the eye of people staring but obviously trying not to, busily returning to whatever they were doing trying to make the transition seemless as we do when we're caught bang to rights! In the past I would have been very self conscious, now I was just glad to be alive and able to go out socially, let them stare, may the force be with you as Yoda would say!

Chapter Five

The In-between Times

Financial Meltdown – Thank God for Social Workers, family and friends.

Whilst in theory I could hide away in a hospital bed in my morphine/antibiotic/infection fuelled haze, the periods of lucidity brought me into a somewhat harsh reality : unemployed and house up for sale in the worse recession since the 1930's, a mortgage to pay, massive overdraft and credit card debts, nothing much to stress about then! Six months previously I had been in a well paid job and whilst finance could be tight on occasions, it was nothing compared to this predicament, this was serious!

When we are at our lowest ebb it appears that everything about us is negative. A lottery win for a depressed person would probably be met with a response such as "now I'll be plagued with begging letters, life will be full of harassment from now on" or statements of a similar ilk. So, there I was, the anaemic leukaemic, mulling over the fact that no one would want to employ me given my dodgy sickness record, we could lose the house and I was generally struggling to see any light at the end of the leukaemia filled tunnel. Facing death does tend to put things in perspective however. For those losing the will to live due to the depressing scenario, stick with me, there is always hope!

Social workers are a much maligned and misrepresented breed of people. Stereotypical images usually portray a long haired, bearded, middle aged hippy type character with leather jacket (and that's just the women). Having worked with a number over recent years I have to say that they are a special breed of person. To take on the role they undertake with members of society usually at their most vulnerable with little reward in terms of positive feedback requires a special type of person. Their task is being made increasingly difficult by increased bureaucracy and an increased workload. Stress I would imagine is on the essential criteria of their person specification. Through all this, however, a desire to help people genuinely shines through.

I needed help. Some of you may well have drawn that conclusion long since. I needed to minimise any stress in my life as I was convinced that being in such a state financially would not do me any good physically and would certainly prolong my recovery. Having decided that the black cloaked figure with his scythe could leave me alone for a few years, I needed a strategy to take me forward, this included importantly, our finances. My soul mate Sandra would be worse off if I shuttled off so there was another reason to hang around for a bit.

Please step forward Carol, my appointed Social Worker and knightess in shining armour who came to my rescue. There were a team of dedicated social workers attached to haematological services at the Royal Victoria Hospital thankfully, and I am sure that they are kept fully occupied. So, Carol visited a pathetic looking and highly emotional specimen primarily to see how I could be helped financially.

With help from her colleague Alan (an ageing hippie who sported a superb beard, the world would be a better place if there were more Alan's in it) I applied for Employment Support Allowance or ESA, here we go again on the short and snappy abbreviation bandwagon. Luckily Carol and Alan sorted out the paperwork due to its complexity and the fact that I now had the attention span of a delirious goldfish.

It is at times like these that the generosity of others in the form of charitable giving and the subsequent practical help such organisations can give is really brought home. Carol applied for grants for me from MacMillan Cancer Care and also the Kay Kendall Leukaemia Fund. I was blessed to receive funds to help with the likes of increased gas and electric bills, wood for our stove and our telephone costs (both land line and mobile calls increased dramatically). To receive such monies at this time was a very humbling experience and I was deeply moved that such organisations existed and were supported so well. I aim to undertake some activities in the future to repay their kindness.

Having never been out of work before, I was in a completely new world, the world of benefits and the DWP, there I go I'm now driving the abbreviation bandwagon, Department of Work and Pensions for the uninitiated. I was to apply for DLA (that is Disability Living Allowance or Degenerate Lounging Allowance as one of our friends jokingly referred to it). Again, Carol completed the paperwork and I was awarded this which eased the financial burden. It was a strange experience in that I immediately felt guilty on receiving this benefit. It took a while and much reassurance from people around me to lessen this feeling. Mum kindly cleared my credit card debt and in the meantime my uncle thankfully responded to a request for a loan to help us through these lean times. I was truly blessed to have such people to call on. We also applied for a mortgage holiday. I had a vision of the title deeds to the house sunning themselves in a deckchair on a beach in the Caribbean. So we had six months breathing space. We were warned that payments would increase on their return, plus there was a £99 fee for stopping payments for six months (to me this sounded like an expensive press of a button on some computer keyboard in the deepest recesses of some mortgage department). As an aside, did you know that mortgages are the biggest scam in the financial world ? They lend us money that doesn't exist and charge us interest on it. Nice one !

So the outlook grew much less bleak thanks to a number of people who helped us along the way at this time. Sometimes, experiencing such vulnerability opens you to accepting the help and love of others, and, highlights the fact that this world isn't such a bad place after all. It also helped me to put aspects of life into perspective, as long as I was clothed, fed and had somewhere to lay my bald head at nights, what was there to really worry about ?

The Homecoming and An Uncertain Doglet

The parole board had agreed I was to be freed on Christmas Eve, a wonderful Christmas present. I had been in hospital since 27th November, a date now etched on my mind, it felt like a lifetime. I was clear of infection but did feel very weak, so much so that a trip to the toilet and back was a major achievement. Having been a complete technophobe prior to becoming ill, I was now a text demon. As soon as I was given the ok to go home the texts began, plans were made. Janice, my sister and her husband Mike had come up to Cumbria along with my niece Caitlin to stay with mum and dad. Mike kindly offered to bring me home, relieving Sandra of the stress of driving.

Christmas Eve dawned, though it didn't feel very Christmassy as you will probably appreciate. There was a distinct purpose for getting up and showered and dressed this particular morning though, I was going home. I had to start early as there was packing to do and with my energy being the equivalent of a gnat on valium I needed hours to do what would take normal folk seconds or minutes at most. I was a trainee leukaemic at this stage, but portraying the role very well on reflection.

I was in conflict to a certain extent. Whereas I couldn't wait to leave the place at least I was safe and being looked after where even a sneeze was treated seriously. How would I get on at home? I was given in depth advice and instructions on what I needed to do if I became unwell. This was serious stuff, I had seen people on the ward fine one minute, having a visit from the scythe wielding spectre the next. Overall, my looking forward to freedom and becoming de-institutionalised overrode what anxieties I had.

My medication arrived from the pharmacy, three bags full of goodies. Michelle, one of the nurses, went through the list of what I had to take and when. Momentarily I thought of a new career in drug dealing, there was some moneys worth in those bags. I decided against this though, my need for those bags and their contents was greater, especially for the morphine as I was still walking like an apprentice cowboy who hadn't been out of the saddle for a month. The pain in my legs was still present. I was set to go, just my chauffeur and new carer to arrive and I would be free. Wait a minute though, there was a dilemma. What do I say to the other inmates as I left ? Tricky situation, tact and diplomacy were warranted. "Live long and prosper" from Mr Spock in the Star Trek films was probably inappropriate. "Hope not to see you soon" may have worked for some, not for those playing cards with the guy with his scythe though. I decided on "Take care I hope all goes well". It seemed to work, the potentially more sensitive interactions were avoided due to those individuals being asleep. Thus I crept out dishing out bags of crisps, orange juice and Lucozade™ like some anaemic, spectral version of Father Christmas.

I had a wheelchair ride to the main entrance, such was my fitness level. There it was, the gaping archway, the main entrance of the hospital and.............my route to freedom and fresh air, well as fresh as it gets in a city centre, carbon monoxide never smelt so good. The view of traffic, buildings, flower beds, the park over the road, all were magnificent, the equivalent to a pint of beer for the ex-con after a thirty year stretch. It got better as we left Newcastle, green fields, I was getting emotional, it was all too much!

So here I was in unfamiliar clothing (a hooded top and thick tracksuit bottoms) complete with hat hiding a shiny dome, Yoda had arrived home, well at mum and dads' at any rate where my sister and niece were also part of the welcoming committee. Toby our doggy companion came running up the hall unsure who I was. He faintly wagged, ears back, meaning the doggy equivalent of "I'm not so sure about who this dude is". I smelt of hospital, had different clothes no hair and a ghost like complexion. No wonder the poor lad was confused. It would be a few weeks before I would be the pack leader again! The family went through the usual polite conversation and Sandra and I then headed back home to our house, our bed, our wood burning stove, our toilet. I wept.

Mr Gut Bucket and The Steroids

Sounds like a pop group doesn't it. I have visions of them playing a smoke filled jazz club…nice…easy. Dexamethasone. It's a mouthful certainly, one chap on the ward with ill fitting dentures tried to say it without a safety net and it took an hour and a half to locate his teeth, three beds away ! Given it's name one would expect a large tablet, in reality mine was the tiniest white pill you could imagine. It is a steroid. The majority of people frown at the word and mutterings usually follow along the lines of "You wouldn't catch me taking those things", "You don't want to be on those things" or things of similar ilk. Too true I didn't want to be on anything but where pain was involved I would take whatever was on offer. My trouble lay in my right arm, damaged in the early days of chemotherapy and causing me severe pain so much so that I couldn't use my arm or bend it without much grimacing and my phantom hair standing on end.

Steroids are amazing drugs. In the first instance my introduction to them was to act as an anti-inflammatory drug for my arm, it worked a treat. The pain went and although I was unable to have a full range of movement I could sleep through the night undisturbed. It seems however that with every drug there are drawbacks lurking in the background in the form of side effects. Yes, the old side effect ploy, fix one thing and create another problem elsewhere, hopefully not as severe as the original reason for treatment. Still with me ? I'm glad you are I think I've lost the plot.

So with my supply of Dexamethasone I was discharged home and was under instructions to take them only when absolutely necessary. I had the grand total of three tablets. What were these things ? Side effect number one for me concerned my bowels. The fact that our local water treatment plant was being overhauled and repaired and the side effect of steroid treatment on my bowels was purely coincidental. Going to the loo became an ordeal, I will leave the rest to your own warped imagination. Suffice to say that this led us to carry out a *Which?* style survey of air fresheners and toilet cleaners. None really stood out, enough said!

Side effect number two for me concerned my appetite. Steroids can lead to weight gain. When I say increased, bear in mind that I had been eating minimal amounts whilst undergoing chemotherapy, it became insatiable. I would hover around the kitchen almost salivating at meal times like a dog with worms. I would eat voraciously. One breakfast, for example consisted of 6 rashers of bacon, 2 eggs, a tin of beans and half a loaf. I would be hungry again two hours later ! I saw now why they only gave me three tablets, these were potent wee beasties. Thus for a few weeks I became Mr Gut Bucket, putting on over a stone in just a few weeks. In addition to the effect of the steroids it was as if my body was craving protein and somehow preparing me for the next slimming session in the form of chemotherapy. I began to wonder if liposuction would be available as part of my treatment plan then remembered that my appointment with the slimming club was imminent.

Infection Paranoia and a Dodgy Thermometer

Having no immune system is a sobering experience. From an early stage after diagnosis the leukaemic is constantly reminded of the need to stay well in between treatments and to report any out of the ordinary symptoms. On discharge I was given an information card which stated that I must report any of the following symptoms immediately.

- A raised temperature (that is Above 38c at any time or Above 37.5c at any two readings taken an hour or more apart)
- Uncontrolled shivering or shaking
- A sore throat
- Diarrhoea
- A cough or shortness of breath
- Discomfort or pain on passing urine
- A rash
- Bruising or bleeding for no apparent reason
- For patients with a long line – redness, pain, swelling or discharge from the exit site

As you can see this was quite scary stuff. With no immune system – I do not over exaggerate here, your white cell count goes down to zero, you can't get much lower than that – you therefore have to rely on antibiotics, anti-viral and/or anti-fungal drugs to do their stuff and fight anything you pick up in terms of infection. Hygiene becomes critical, hand washing and food hygiene take on a really major focus. In between treatments I was given all three types of drugs to take prophylactically (that is as a preventative measure, impressed?). Other advice forthcoming was to avoid contact with anyone who had an infection and to avoid going into places where there were huge numbers of people. I became a hermit. Any visitors had to be vetted by my carer Sandra before admittance to the house!

Just how important this information is was highlighted to me after a week or so into my first chemotherapy treatment. The chap opposite me began with a raised temperature of 38.2 when taken by the nurses at their regular observations during late evening. This chap had an infection in his Hickman Line®, the tube that goes into the chest to deliver the chemotherapy drugs. Within 30 minutes his temperature reached 40c and he was uncontrollably shivering, things were getting serious and he was rushed off to ITU (the Intensive Therapy Unit) where his line was taken out and another inserted in his neck as his other veins were collapsing and he needed intravenous antibiotics urgently. His family feared the worst, a priest was sent for, this was serious stuff. All this within 30 minutes! When things happen they do so rapidly. Sitting at home thinking 'this temperature will go if I pop a Paracetamol' was not an option as far as I was concerned. One sneeze and I would be on the phone!

So before my first release we needed a tympanic thermometer (one that you stick in the ear, the type they used on the ward). Sandra found one in Carlisle at the pharmacy over the road from where she works "we don't usually stock these, don't know why it was ordered" thus spoke the pharmacist. We were definitely being looked after. It was purchased at a bargain price, we were armed to commence the regular testing and appease the paranoia somewhat.

It was agreed with Dr O'Brien, my consultant in Carlisle that I would have a bed in Carlisle at the Infirmary should I need one in between planned visits to Newcastle. I did, unfortunately require 3 unplanned admissions due to what appeared to be the beginning of some infection. I received excellent care on Larch D ward at the Infirmary. We did discover that our thermometer was slightly out when compared to the ward thermometer. A replacement was duly sent for and all was well. The usual protocol was to have 72 hours of antibiotics therapy and if all was well, I would toddle off home.

The impact of the chemotherapy treatment on the body is enormous. Here I was at home, anaemic and subsequently Lethargic Lenny, a lowered platelet count hence nosebleeds, the effect of the chemotherapy drugs leading to bone and muscular aches, my problem was I felt lousy, how do I tell if I feel different? The thermometer was the key, hourly checks from waking till night and during the night if I awoke. Initially it was a part of the routine and a novelty. I began to loathe the process and resented the fact that I may have to go back to hospital. I was not a happy bunny! There were positives though, I had my own room when admitted to the

Cumberland Infirmary, pleasant nursing staff and a view, yes a longed for view to the Lake District fells. Above all, I was still alive and kicking.

The Impatient Outpatient

A diagnosis of any form of cancer takes over your life, leukaemia is no different. A prolonged episode of in-patient treatment, out-patient clinics, blood and platelet transfusions and constant self monitoring follows diagnosis. Any time for self indulgence is strictly limited, any plans for such usually ended up cancelled due to Lethargic Lenny or some other such affliction taking hold.

Outpatient clinics were a regular occurrence, usually three times per week whilst I was neutropenic (that is my neutrophils the soldiers of my immune system had gone on holiday), this to monitor my white cell count and importantly my haemoglobin and platelet levels to ensure I received transfusions when the levels began to fall into the dangerous zone. Fortunately I attended these at the Cumberland Infirmary in Carlisle as opposed to the 150 mile round trip to Newcastle.

Rumour has it that the new building at the Infirmary, one of the first of the governments Private Finance Initiative or PFI (away we go again) was designed by an architect who has designed airports. Certainly all it would take would be a few wheeled cases and you could be looking for your flight departure as opposed to your outpatient clinic. The Atrium, as it is known, is a huge area, the wards small and cramped, mmm. The classic is that the orthopaedic clinic dealing with all the fractures and such like is the furthest point from the main entrance, keeps the folks on crutches fit though ! The architects, Bodgit, Leggit and Scarper Associates now have their main office in Smugsville. Bitter and twisted, me?

Dr O'Brien, my consultant, held his clinics on the lower ground floor, next door to the mortuary! Fortunately he never used the phrase 'Just pop next door for a moment'. This location was the equivalent of a country mile for the anaemic leukaemic. Sandra would drop me off at the front of the airport, sorry, hospital and I would wend my way thither, often being overtaken by 90 year old ladies with zimmer frames or people on crutches, such was my fitness. I was forced to use the lifts, stairs were a no go area. For those unfamiliar with hospital lifts I wouldn't say the wait for one was long but there were generally two or three skeletons along with long bearded men milling about. Lifts are a strange environment, nobody speaks, eye contact is nil and it appears compulsory to stare at either the ceiling or your shoes. Conversations in full flow when the lift arrives are cut short only to resume as the lift doors open on the destination floor. We are funny things us humans.

There were two consulting rooms for Dr O'Brien to use and outside these was a small waiting area with the usual faded magazines from 1997. Adjacent to this waiting area was a main thoroughfare for staff which led to a secure part of the hospital through a door which was operated by a swipe card system. On average every 30 seconds or so a group or an individual would hurry past and swipe their card(s) to enter.

Dr O'Brien operated an excellent system which meant a minimal wait at his clinic. He would take blood and the results would be through between 5 and 10 minutes later. Impressive service, the last thing I wanted when I was feeling rough was a long wait. It was during the time spent in the waiting area I used to play a game I called 'Catch Eye and Smile'. The thoroughfare of staff brought people of all shapes, sizes and ages past the waiting area. It was like being on display at the zoo, I imagined a sign "Anaemic Leukaemic – Ghastlius Horriblus, this fine example was discovered in the wolds of Cumbria...." which they could read as they wandered past. I began to reverse the trend and stare back, a bit like the orang-utans do in the zoo in between cigars and champagne back in their private quarters. Some people were clearly uncomfortable with this and immediately would look away, some smiled back guiltily, yet others would start fiddling with keys or swipe card. One poor man spilt his coffee as he failed to realise the door he was going through was locked. Some light mirth thus ensued.

There are certain advantages to serious illness, sometimes unlooked for. I now know all the staff at the GP surgery and similarly on the wards in Newcastle and Carlisle where I had my treatment including my numerous transfusions. Above this though, was the status that goes with such a serious illness, as highlighted by the following scenario. After my treatment had finished I arranged to go to see my GP as I felt rough and had also developed a rash over my torso. The walk from the car park into the surgery did me no favours, I was out of breath and wheezed at the receptionist before unfortunately taking a seat next to an older gentleman who, it was soon established, clearly didn't get out much and made up for his deficit in social contact on his visit to the doctors. Normally I would have obliged and engaged in a lengthy conversation. This day, however was different. He began by telling me he thought he had hay fever and went on to describe his symptoms in great detail to me as if I were his GP – the whole waiting room listened on, glad they were not in the hot seat I had chosen. After a ten minute oratory I was given my opportunity, "What you ere for then?". "Leukaemia", I offered. The conversation halted and there was much shuffling and coughing in the waiting area. One nil and game over thought I. I was in the higher echelons of the illness league. If you've got it, flaunt it as the saying goes !

Build Me Up, Knock Me Down – A Tale Of Mr Grumpy

When diagnosed with a serious illness such as leukaemia you naturally expect to feel unwell, the chemotherapy itself adds to this leaving a pathetic looking specimen in my case. This, I would tell myself, is par for the course, the black cloaked spectre and his scythe never visit the wrong one! Having said that I have visions of him being given a Sat Nav and ending up in a river somewhere finishing up with a rusty scythe. So, after the first batch of chemotherapy I was sent home complete with infection paranoia and having had an injection of G-CSF. This is designed to stimulate the production of neutrophils and to reduce the duration of chemotherapy induced neutropenia (little or no immune system) and thereby reduce the risk of infection, which by now you know to be life threatening. Unfortunately this injection led me to experience severe bone pain and led me to start dabbling with opiates again. Nurse.....!

After a few weeks at home, I was improving, I looked and felt less like a corpse. My immune system returned, my haemoglobin and platelets returned to near normal levels. I could go out, I could walk short distances, I could live a little. My taste returned and I had an appetite. The stairs were no longer like part of assault course to gain entry into the parachute regiment. What we all tend to take for granted, I could start to do again, even drying dishes became a source of major achievement and pleasure. This was a short term phenomena though and soon returned to being a chore.

So there I was, life beginning to flow in my bones again, just in time for......the next chemotherapy session and subsequent hospital stay. I would be greeted by nursing staff on the ward with "Don't you look well, we'll soon change that". It was funny the first time, by the end it resulted in much teeth grinding and muttering. This was the hardest part of the whole leukaemia saga, the planned suffering. I became a grump. Those close to me could detect a change about two or three days before admission. I would become withdrawn and 'tetchy'. The journeys across to Newcastle would be generally in silence. Sometimes I was given a reprieve if there was no bed available. I would have cart wheeled down the hallway but I could never do cartwheels, usually ending up in a crumbled heap with the PE teacher trying not to laugh and in any case my energy levels weren't really up to that. Having had a taste of freedom, the incarceration was hard to take. Somehow I battled through.

Chapter Six

Reflections

Beware – You Are Now Entering The Emotional Zone

For those who find the emotional side of life difficult to deal with, I suggest you have a number of options. Firstly, skip this chapter altogether, secondly stick your fingers in your ears whilst reading this or thirdly read it with intrigue and an open mind to discover how one of your colleagues in the game of life experienced the enigma that is cancer. For those who enjoy an emotion evoking diatribe, read on and enjoy.

It has to be said that with this chapter I become more serious as it is an opportunity to reflect on how I made it to this point. I aim to examine what helped, what didn't and above all the emotional drain that cancer can bring. Depressed ? You may be.....Given hope ?....you will be.

Unsung Heroes

In some respects, spouses, partners, those we are close to, have as much to deal with, if not more, than the sufferer themselves. Sandra, my dear soul mate was no exception. Practically it meant an increased workload in terms of housework, the usual domestic chores of washing, ironing, shopping and cleaning were all laid squarely at her door. This alongside her usual part time job, visiting me on her days off, meant a stressful juggling act.

Initially, during the days following diagnosis was the difficult task of telling family, friends, work colleagues past and present along with neighbours what had taken place. Imagine all the emotional upheaval that goes with this process. This again, was down to Sandra and it was no wonder that within a few days she was emotionally drained but hid this well from me, or so she thought! The closer the relationship, the more heightened the emotions, driven primarily through fear of loss. In some ways it was almost like a bereavement in terms of ringing round and the repeated emotional strain of relaying the tale of the anaemic leukaemic which never seemed to lessen in terms of psychological pain the more it was told in those early days. In other ways it was like a bereavement in that an old part of me died, a new and stronger version sits writing this.

To watch someone you love suffer and have the potential scenario of losing them is a difficult situation to go through. It is no wonder that Sandra needed support herself. We were blessed to have family, friends and neighbours who could provide this where I could not. It is, at times such as this when we reflect that we chose well when forming the friendships we did in the past. True friends know us at a deep level, they know when we need space and when we are in need of that shoulder on which to blubber. Fortunately we had such people in our lives.

Hello my Friend, Goodbye.......

People come and go out of our lives, that appears to be the way of our journeys through life. Sometimes, even the briefest liaison with another person seems to be pre-planned. So it was with Jeff. I had arrived in Newcastle and had my diagnosis confirmed, Sandra had been sent on her way to negotiate the journey back to Cumbria via a tour of Tyneside. I was awaiting a bed and had been ushered into the patients lounge in which sat Jeff. We got talking, he had been diagnosed a couple of months previously and was quite upbeat despite this. On finding out about my predicament he proceeded to give me reassurance and hope and allay any fears I had over the chemotherapy. I couldn't have asked for more at that moment in time, entering a whole new world I was given my own personal tour guide.

Our paths crossed on a number of occasions either on the ward or at outpatient clinics. It was during these meetings that I discovered a common bond between everyone on the ward and those in the clinics. It is as if some deep understanding occurs, true some did not want to speak, even so a look into their eyes would reflect back this understanding, this sharing of experience, perhaps this facing of death. The last time I met Jeff was at an outpatient appointment in Newcastle. I was having a bone marrow biopsy prior to seeing my Consultant, Jeff was having a blood transfusion, a common sight for us leukaemics. On going over to talk to him we exchanged the usual pleasantries, Jeff was not his usual self. He announced that the doctors had said they could do no more for him. His condition was terminal.

I drew on my nursing experience and told him that whatever happened he would be alright, something I firmly believe. Death for me is a gateway into a different experience and reality. I did not see Jeff again and do know that he has now passed over. I thank his soul for what he did for me with his words of comfort. There were other people I met on the wards who similarly came and went. I learnt not to ask too many questions of the nursing staff, firstly because of them being bound by rules of confidentiality, secondly I didn't really want to know for my own sake. If I didn't know that they had died officially, there was still hope. The more people died the greater the sense of ones own mortality and the leukaemia begins to turn into an ever increasing threat. This was why I avoided studying percentages in terms of survival rates lest I should turn a potentially negative outcome into reality and cause additional stress which I believed created the problem in the first place. To all that have come and gone during my brief cancer journey, may their souls rest in peace and may their loved ones find strength, courage and peace.

Recovery (Survivorship)

Lance Armstrong the elite athletic cyclist and multiple Tour de France winner suffered testicular cancer and had a brutal regime of chemotherapy, overcoming a 2% chance of survival. In his book *"It's Not About The Bike"* , he describes a phenomenon he calls survivorship. This is the period after treatment when you find yourself in remission but no longer a cancer 'patient'.

On reading Armstrong's book immediately after diagnosis I struggled to grasp this concept of survivorship thinking that whatever happened to me I wouldn't let this affect me to the same degree, that is becoming depressed with nothing to do or aim for. A foolish notion as it turned out that this period post treatment is probably the hardest to cope with. Surely the moment the Consultant tells you that "Your blood results are fine, there is no need to see you now for a month, cheerio", , this should be a moment which gives cause for rejoicing. The removal of my Hickman Line® from my chest was a moment I had described over the previous months as my ultimate goal, this would be the cause of celebration and a major hurdle in my battle against the foe that was leukaemia. How was it then that these major milestones passed with a laissez faire attitude from myself.

From the moment I was given the diagnosis, that is I became a leukaemic, a patient, my mind was focused more on short term goals. I was a regular in-patient and out-patient , I had a role within society and a clear path to follow in terms of my treatment plan agreed with Professor Jackson and his colleagues. My goals would change from week to week. The end of the treatment is a sobering experience. Yes, you begin to feel better physically, albeit over a longer period than anticipated, the psychological trauma, however, appears to kick in at this point, my path suddenly ended at a cliff top.

Reflecting upon this period is difficult as it was a period I would rather not reflect upon. Part of our psyche, I would argue, engages us in some kind of self analysis as to what is happening and why in an attempt to rationalise why after coming through months of suffering and torment I reach a point where I wonder what was the point. I felt that I should have gone early on and saved myself all the suffering. Thus my psychoanalyst alter ego began the task of unravelling the potential reasoning for my lowered mood.

Firstly I lost a focus, a goal. During treatment I had little goals to aim for along the way, now what was there ? Physical recovery, I was informed, would be at least six months. I imagined mistakenly, that my progress would continue at the pace it had between treatments. It appeared that the cumulative effect of the chemotherapy resulted in me hitting a plateau whereafter progress in terms of energetic recovery becomes tediously slow. The four walls of the hospital are swapped for those of home. I was adrift in the sea of recovery without a paddle.

Secondly, I lost my role as an active patient. Although my lack of hair, eyebrows and facial growth meant I still looked the part, this soon went. A ruddy complexion and renewed hair growth was met with "Don't you look well", soon followed by "When are you back at work ?" I was hanging on to the sick role by my finger nails, I was uncomfortable in this no-man's land. The lack of contact with the health service also served to highlight my lack of a role – nobody wanted me. I would seek out confirmation from my GP whenever the opportunity arose to see him, I was still ill wasn't I ?

Thirdly, this period post treatment gave me time to think. Cogitating about the treatment and all the issues surrounding it, major issues usually, suddenly had come to an end, leaving me with a huge amount to sit and think about. Initially this was a time to reflect upon what had actually happened, my skirt with death, the reserves I had used up in the process and the realisation that I was drained. Like the marathon runner who has just crossed the line, I needed to draw breath and recover. Reality began to stare me in the face. The spectre of the future came to haunt me – unemployed, financial difficulties, struggling to do much, where do I go from here ? Was it all really worth it ?

I was left in a state of limbo where a sword dangled over me. The threat of the leukaemia returning was an ever present spectre at my shoulder from waking until sleep took hold each night. From day one I had been told that 'remission' was not the same as 'cured'. Like an ever increasing brooding presence the risk was there whatever I thought or did – fact.

My mood plummeted. My behaviour changed. I would stay in bed under the guise of tiredness, there was tiredness but also the desire not to face the world. What was the point ? I lazed about the house. I was on a short fuse. I didn't want to talk to anyone, Sandra had to deflect phone calls and visits to the house under the "He's not so good at the moment" ploy. My self esteem went. I was a wretched and pathetic specimen of self piteous misery. Cancer had finally got to me.

To Transplant or Not To Transplant That was The Question !

From diagnosis day when the word transplant was first mentioned my gut reaction was to avoid this at all costs. My head and the fear of dying and my deep inner survival driver went along with the idea as the route to self preservation. There was, however, an initial compromise, I would have a transplant if there was no other option, that is I would die without one. So the wheels of the transplant machine sprang into action, my sister, Janice agreed to be a donor and was tested on a visit to the ward and was subsequently found to be a perfect match.

After two bouts of chemotherapy and going into remission after both of these I was fast approaching a crossroads, a time to reflect on my treatment and determine what future treatment I needed. The medical team were erring on the side of a transplant. I, on the other hand had been doing a bit of research into transplants myself. There was information available in pamphlet form such as "Understanding Stem Cell and Bone Marrow Transplants", a booklet produced by the charity Cancerbackup. I must stress at this point that anyone reading this prior to making a decision regarding a bone marrow transplant should not base their decision solely on my writings here. I am merely explaining the rationale for my decision to decline a transplant as I interpreted what I read and saw happening around me. There are lots of sources of information available, both written and human, notably the medical profession in whose care you entrust your life on which to base your own decision.

As with any type of medical procedure there are risks involved. Stem cell and bone marrow transplants are no exception. I would have had a stem cell transplant, this would involve a 3-4 hour procedure during which the donor (in this case Janice my sister) would have a drip put in a vein in each arm. Blood would be taken from one arm through the drip and collected in a machine called a stem cell separator, its clever stuff this! This separator spins the blood to separate out the stem cells. These are collected and the remaining blood is returned to the donor through the other arm. Before the collected stem cells would be given to me, however, I would have had a course of 'High Dose Chemotherapy' ! "This treatment is both physically and emotionally demanding. You may need to stay in hospital for up to four weeks or longer, and there may be times when you feel very unwell", so said the pamphlet. At least they tell it how it really is.

Then we have the risks associated with a transplant:-

- Graft Failure: Sometimes the transplant of stem cells fails to make the bone marrow produce enough new blood cells leading to repeated infections, bruising, bleeding and anaemia.
- Veno-Occlusive Disease: The high dose chemotherapy can cause a serious liver problem in which the blood in the liver become swollen and blocked.
- Graft-versus-Host-Disease: This occurs where transplant is from a donor. There is the possibility that the new cells (the graft) will react against the recipients tissues (the host). It is generally mild but can be life threatening in some people where it mainly affects the skin, the gut (stomach and bowel) and the liver.
- After high dose chemotherapy treatment there is the risk of possible life threatening infections and

bleeding. The recipient of a transplant would usually be nursed in isolation in a cubicle within the ward.
- Death: Some people die during the procedure.

It must be said that managing such risks is where the skill and expertise of the medical team come into play.

It is widely acknowledged that a transplant is a traumatic experience and can often lead to anxiety and depression. Certainly my observations on the ward would bear this out, where strong individuals appeared to increasingly suffer psychologically as the treatment progressed. Mention must also be made of the relationship between the donor and the recipient. Where the donor is known, as in a sibling, to receive the gift of life from someone will, undoubtedly, leave the recipient in debt to that person. Where it fails there is also the possibility of blame rearing its head. What I am trying to say is that it may well test the strongest of family relationships.

In certain scenarios a transplant may be the only option available to sustain life, in which case all the above merely become things to look out for, or experience during the treatment. I was fortunate in that I was classed as a 'middle risk' patient. I could choose, although having said that the initial thoughts of the medical team was to transplant. It is often hard to go against such advice. On this matter though, my mind was made up, even before I had the opportunity to discuss it with Professor Jackson. Having observed transplant recipients on the ward and read the literature I decided that even if it meant dying prematurely, I would rather have a few months with a good quality of life than the next few years continuing to suffer. I had suffered for two years to this point, enough was enough.

Many will find this a bizarre decision and question my sanity at this point. I would respond with the fact that this was my body, my life and my future. I have that right to choose even if it seems a strange decision. I know a number of people who have had transplants and regretted doing so. For me, the length of time in isolation and for recovery would have resulted in major psychological distress. I am glad I made the decision I did. In the end, Professor Jackson acknowledged that he was unsure what he would have done in my situation. It is a balancing act. The negatives were the fact that I had been ill for so long prior to diagnosis along with my cytogenetics which put me into the medium risk category. (Cytogenetics relates to the chromosomes which are made up of genes, these control the activities of the cell.) By testing bone marrow with a cytogenetic test, changes in structure can be detected and treatment regimes determined. This was where the doctors earned their corn. The positives, there are always positives, were the fact that I was "young and extremely fit", Professor Jackson's words not mine, alongside the fact that I had responded well by going into remission after each treatment of chemotherapy. It was my shout basically and I remain glad that I chose as I did. Time will tell whether I was right or not but it cannot be denied that I am blessed with each day given to me and am enjoying life as never before. I will cover the concept of transplants in Part Two as I believe it is a procedure with more to it than just the physical act of the transplant and can have profound psychological effects on the recipient.

How Did I Cope ?

It has been an interesting exercise to reflect on what got me through the last two years. I have to acknowledge that prior to diagnosis I did not cope particularly well and was very close to leaving this world of my own volition. It would appear that a lack of hope for the future at this time found me having increasing difficulty to battle through the symptoms I was experiencing. The lack of a specific diagnosis at this point led to a kind of self blaming scenario along with depression as a result of the suffering I was experiencing. Being diagnosed was a relief. I was not imagining all the symptoms I had suffered and am sure that a number of people believed they were psychosomatic.

How then did I cope after diagnosis ? There are a number of factors which helped me through. Firstly, I have a belief system. I believe in God and that we are spiritual beings having a human experience which can be difficult and challenging at times. I also believe we have incarnated many times before and that we are given the opportunity with each lifetime to develop our souls through lessons we learn as human beings. Prior to arriving on the planet we plan such opportunities. As such, death is merely going through a doorway into another reality or dimension. When first diagnosed I did not think that I was going to die, something deep within me told me that I still had unfinished business. Our world is set to experience major change, for the better I hasten to add, over the coming years, somehow I know I am to be involved in this process.

Being a rational type of person I asked the question I am sure all of us ask in such circumstances, *"Why me?"* To answer this let us look at all the positives that came out of this life changing event. I had a physical deep clean. My view of my body changed. I now treat it with more respect, ensuring I eat healthily and do not put it under undue stress. It is difficult for many people to understand but leukaemia has been a blessing for me, a kind of wake up call which gave me a healing space and time out of my previous role and its associated daily stressors. In some ways my hand has been forced to get out of that situation and review my life and the future.

I have gained new strength. Facing death certainly puts things into perspective. My self confidence has soared, after all, what is there to worry about now ? My outlook has subsequently changed, I am blessed to have food on a daily basis, to have a roof over my head and to be able to wander in our beautiful countryside. I see the world with new eyes, almost that of a newborn. This Spring has been the best ever for me. Appreciation and gratitude are daily companions for me now. The only way is up.

The support I have received has been overwhelming and often unlooked for. I have a box full of cards, letters and messages from family and friends and work colleagues past and present whom I count as friends. I had books and magazines as gifts to help me survive the long days along with clothes, a DVD player, an iPod and a Sony Walkman. I was introduced to Radio Newcastle which although very culturally different from my local Radio Cumbria did keep me going through many a long day and night. I had arrived as far as technology was concerned ! In terms of support, I include the therapies and healings I received on request and often volunteered on behalf of the therapists, to whom I am deeply grateful. This confidence in complementary medicine and in the medical team I was in the care of was a further reason for my ability to cope.

I set myself daily goals which were realistic and that I could achieve. The way I felt each day varied so much that it would be unrealistic and psychologically damaging to plan too far ahead. Whilst on the ward in the early days of treatment a walk down to the end of the ward corridor was something I could only manage on a few occasions. I would duly plan this when I felt able to do it and not push my body too far. I learnt that doing nothing was a part of the healing process and can be set as a goal on the days where my energy levels were particularly low. In this way I was able to exert some sort of control over my daily routine.

I was shown courage on the ward from others. There were people who inspired me to carry on. One individual had been unwell for two years, had battled through two stem cell transplants and yet faced each day despite its guaranteed suffering with grace and humour. I gained strength from such individuals. There are amazing people on earth at this time. Part of my personality is stubborn and a deep determination set in from an early stage that I would survive. I have run half marathons in the past where physical pain is overcome through mental strength. This was no different.

Let me finally state that overall, the leukaemia has given me a lot of positive aspects of which I am grateful. That said, however, it should not detract from the fact that there are parts of the experience which are unpleasant and grim. It is at these times of both physical and psychological suffering that we are given the opportunity to dig deep into those recesses reserved for such occasions and demonstrate our strength.

Highs and Lows

Anyone familiar with employee appraisal systems will be aware of the need to start with 'the areas that need improvement' or 'weaknesses' in pre-nanny state language. After this come the positives, what we are good at and excel at. Thus to follow a similar pattern I will duly start with the low points of my journey through leukaemia. I suggest you save this until you are having a good day !

Before diagnosis there was a period of time when I was ready to depart this life. Not exactly making plans as we say in the psychiatric trade, but not far off. The itching, lack of sleep, the juggling act trying to keep going at work, all became too much. After diagnosis there were similar times. The worst in terms of treatment was probably the third period as an in-patient during which time I spent 24 hours a day attached to a drip delivering chemotherapy for five days. I felt awful both physically and psychologically. This was the time that I nearly gave up and was prepared to throw in the towel, by this I mean rejecting that and any further treatment, suffering the consequences, even if this meant death. Somehow, I got through though. Similar feelings were evident prior to the second and third planned admissions for treatment. I knew what to expect and from feeling pretty good, physically you enter hospital only to be made poorly again.

The lowest point of all surprisingly came after all the treatment had finished. I was left in a no-mans land, I was no longer an active patient, I had no role in society and it also gave me a lot of time to think and reflect on the past months and the fact that I had just come through a life threatening illness. My mood dropped like a stone. Whereas I should have felt like celebrating when back in remission and at having my Hickman Line® removed, I would weep at the drop of a hat. Time is a healer, and within a few weeks of reflection I am back on top form. Apparently this is recognised as normal by the medical profession, it is unfortunate there is no active follow up in terms of psychological support at this time.

So, now that you're feeling pretty depressed let me lift you with tales of the high points along the road. The first came in the discharge home on Christmas Eve, this after a four week spell in hospital after my initial diagnosis. Tears were of joy. Secondly I was able to get out for a semi-serious walk up one of our small fells locally. This was in between the second and third chemotherapy treatments and was something I had dreamed of doing whilst lying in a hospital bed. To smell the heather and see the view from the top was just amazing. Similarly at this time we were able to go out for a pub meal within the Lake District. Just to be able to go out socially after being a semi-hermit for so long was fantastic. These things gave me additional strength and determination to go on, which I did and have.

Each day is a blessing. Before leukaemia (or BL if you want to make it catchy again) I would go through the usual drudgery of routine that was life. Now I welcome each day, look forward to the opportunities that each day will bring. I changed as a person. It is strange to say but leukaemia did me a favour. I woke up, I was tested and am the stronger for it.I hope you now feel buoyant !

Part Two

A Simple Man's Guide to Cancer, The Universe and Everything

"No problem can be solved by the same consciousness that created it"

Albert Einstein

Chapter Seven

Some Basic Beliefs (Is it Me or is it a Mad, Mad World Out There?)

Introduction

Congratulations, you have made it so far with me on my journey through this strange thing we call life and this even stranger phenomenon called cancer. So here I am, writing this still recovering from the poisoning that is chemotherapy. Incidentally, even my Consultant used this phrase in a recent clinic appointment! I have lots of time on my hands to cogitate on events that have taken place regarding my health and still there is the fundamental question I am sure the majority of people ask, Why Me ? There are numerous other questions that come to light when you begin to delve a bit and look at the world slightly differently. Why is cancer on the increase? Why do certain people have what are termed 'Miraculous healings'? Why is there no cure available given all the research and money invested in such? Why so many questions ?

What follows in Part Two will probably test your belief systems, alternatively you will reach the conclusion fairly quickly that I need my bumps felt or that chemotherapy damaged my bonce somehow! What I aim to do is to present information in such a way as to enable you to take responsibility for your own health. As you will see the modern approach to cancer in the Western medical model focuses solely on attacking cancer through what has been termed *'Targeted Therapy'*. What I aim to do in this more serious part of the book is to give you a glimpse of what I see as the bigger picture. I am not saying that the medical system in use is wrong, far from it as it saved my life. All I wish to do is to give you information which is out there but is not well publicised, this in order for you to make an informed choice about treatment should you need it. Unfortunately at this time, one in three of us will. I would suggest that there are certain agendas at play in the system that involves vast sums of money which would like to see the system stay as it is. Having looked at other treatment modalities I do believe that there is no miracle 'cure' for cancer but that it involves many aspects of our lives which the current system fails to address. You may well conclude that this is all rubbish and rely solely on what our current health service can offer you. Indeed it is a sorry state of affairs when lack of finance to engage in the complementary and alternative health scene means that you may be forced to do just this. Certain healings though may well be within the purchasing power of the majority such as the purchase of a self help CD for example.

It is sad that we live in a litigious society and thus I must make it clear that I do not make any claims about cures, at the end of the day it is up to you to use your own discernment and seek healing for yourself in whatever way feels right for you. All I can present is what has happened to me and my belief systems. Thus what I present here is an amalgamation of information which is already out there and working quite effectively for lots of people. I have thus developed a simple model, being a simple soul I thought it quite appropriate! This was developed to try and come up with answers to the old 'Why me?' chestnut. My hope is that the information here may give you food for thought and may well open up new avenues for you. I wish you well.

What I would like to say at this juncture is please do not give your power away and fall into the 'Victim Trap'(or VT if we go continue down the catchy abbreviations route). Please read on with an open mind. I have no hidden agenda other than to help others who are suffering as I did and hopefully prevent people from experiencing such. I am not a professional researcher nor an academic but a simple man who feels that things in the world of healthcare just aren't right and have begun to ask some common sense questions. Material has come into my possession which I was obviously meant to read and as such hopefully provide some answers. Please dare yourself to read on and you may be amazed and even help heal the world and more importantly yourself………

I have pondered (having progressed from musing) on whether to share with you some of my thoughts on the world we live in and have decided that in order for you to understand why I am correlating this information and reaching the conclusions that I do it is necessary for you to know what I think. What I believe in. So here goes.

Some Democracy!

Most people I talk to recognise that we need a change, and by that I don't just mean a change in government. After all, there is no choice politically just another wolf sporting the latest designer sheepskin. Do we really live in a democracy? Yes, we all say, we have a vote. So, how then, when the majority of the country's population did not want a war in Iraq or Afghanistan did we end up there? Mass killings of innocent civilians (up to 27,000 so far, yes that's twenty seven thousand) not to mention the increasing loss of troops who are carrying out the orders of our government. Add to this the legislation which has crept in allegedly to keep us safe from the perceived terrorist threat in similar fashion to the Patriot Act in America and bingo, we are the most spied upon population in the history of the planet. They even know I'm sporting blue undies, not just any undies, but M&S undies, clean on today! You are honoured. Then there is the most recent legislation which means that all our e-mails, texts and internet contacts are all logged and stored for potential use by the authorities. The best thing is we allow it to happen under the guise of keeping us from harm, after all the world is full of terrorists! CCTV, speed cameras, the list goes on. We are even encouraged to join in, shop your neighbour, ring this number now....

We are reliably informed by those in charge that we need them as otherwise anarchy would break out. Really? As Leo Tolstoy, the author of war and peace and pacifist put it

> "....even if the absence of government really meant anarchy in the negative disorderly sense of the word – which is far from being the case – even then no anarchical disorder could be worse than the position to which governments have already led their peoples, and to which they are leading them."

What did George Orwell know when he wrote the now infamous work that is *1984.* It is becoming a reality a bit later than he envisioned but reality nonetheless. Do you feel free? Are you happy with your lot or do you somehow feel you are being controlled and manipulated? I would recommend reading Tom Hodgkinson's *'How To Be Free'* which light heartedly suggests that we were better off in the Middle Ages than we are now with more leisure time and a better quality of life. Despite the humour he sends out a serious message reflecting upon the world we have created for ourselves. The media tells us on a daily basis how horrible the world is, it's a good job we have a government to keep us safe! What utter nonsense. Look at all the good that goes on around us on a daily basis. If they had a 'Good News at Ten' show it would run on into the wee small hours as there would be so much to cover.

What concerns me though is the amount of power we willingly give away to those deemed to be 'in charge', assuming they have our best interests at heart. Certainly there will be a minority that enter the political arena with the interests of others at the heart of what they do. Let us not kid ourselves though that there are a number of very wealthy and powerful organisations which covertly influence our politics not to mention those within the system out for careers and personal gain (just think back to the expenses scandal). Why is it that only a third of the electoral population choose to vote? It may well be that we are becoming increasingly tired of the lies and the playground behaviour that is our so called democratic system ? Wouldn't it be refreshing to hear an MP say the words 'yes' or 'no' or go to such extremes as 'Sorry I don't know'!

For those that think that the decisions are wholly made with our Prime Minister and his cabinet, think again. There are numerous conspiracy theorists who have investigated such things and have shown that power within the world is held in quarters other than the governments of our perceived influential countries. The financial sector, the media, the petrochemical companies, the pharmaceutical companies (more of them later) all hold a powerful sway over global affairs. Do not worry though, we hold enormous power within ourselves. The future from where I am standing looks bright, even brighter than orange.....Change is on the horizon, but more of that later.

We've Done Politics Now For Religion!

The two things we are encouraged not to talk about in company, politics and religion. Well folks, I'm making up for lost time and the good news is that I've 46 and a bit years' worth of keeping it buttoned to make up for. Before I start I do want to make it perfectly clear to you that religions do vast amounts of good and benefit an awful lot of people. I am not against what they stand for, on the contrary if we all followed their core teachings which are all very similar, then the world would indeed be a better place. The essence of each religion, is love, light and spiritual truth. No religion is better or worse than the other, ultimately millions of us use religion as a pathway to God, which has to be beneficial for us and the planet as a whole. Lots of good is done through the practices of religions throughout the world. Go into any community and there will be evidence of this. As usual though, we don't often get to hear about it, after all it's such a bad world we need to keep having this reinforced to us this on a daily basis, don't we?

I was brought up as a Methodist, part of the Christian faith and have met some truly amazing and loving people as a result of this. However, several years ago I began to question what religion was all about. Why for example does the Church in this country steer clear of politics ? We go to war in Iraq, and I ask what would the likes of Jesus or Ghandi have said on the matter? "Don't worry chaps, I'll bend the love thy neighbour rule a bit so as to mean it only applies in this country, will that be ok ?". Don't think so somehow. Other puzzlers were why certain religions appear to display vast material wealth and yet certain members within that faith remain in poverty? Religion, whilst providing spiritual fulfilment along with a concept of social guidance as to what is right and wrong for many people, also has, somewhat inevitably, an aspect of control to it. Why is it that there are human interpretations of original teachings which themselves are very often basically simple such as the 'Love your neighbour as you love yourself' ? In her book *Angel Answers,* Diana Cooper states that

> "Religion is spirit clothed by man. Where there are dogma and rules, pure spirit becomes restricted. Spirituality allows people to be themselves, free to use their intuition, to commune with nature and the spirit world."

It was, perhaps this lack of freedom that I was feeling those several years ago. God is love ultimately, so the big question for me is why does a part of the majority of religions seek to engender fear as part of their teachings. There is the concept of a hell or its equivalent. Why should a loving God send souls for torment ? It just does not make sense. If you were wanting to have an aspect of control over people, however, it makes perfect sense. Fear is the bane of mankind and is preventing us from living to our true potential. In my view even those who have perpetrated horrendous crimes are still loved by God and are lovingly supported to come back in another incarnation to put things right.

People always ask that if God exists why does he allow suffering? We have free will at the end of the day. Disasters for example, are not created by God. Disasters could be interpreted as a natural result of collective human karma. In addition, look at the loving response that usually occurs to such disasters from around the world. We have been given free will to love or destroy, God merely stands back and witnesses our actions. Whatever we do we are still loved, even if our actions create massive amounts of karma and mean we go back to the bottom rung of the spiritual ladder. We are not better than anyone else just because we are on a higher rung, and as we are all part of the One that is God it is in our best interests to help those around us achieve their maximum potential. There lies the route to wisdom. As the old saying goes,

> "Knowledge is knowing that the tomato is a fruit, wisdom is not putting it in a fruit salad!"

Phew! That has been a long time coming and is better out than in. Just a part of me starting to express myself a bit more. Let us move on to look at my view (along with a growing number of people on the planet I hasten to add) of what we humans actually are.

There's More To Us Than Meets The Eye....

When you look in the mirror what do you see. Flesh and bones, our biological bubble that enables our spirit to experience life in human form. For ultimately that is what we are, spirits. We cannot die, we just go from one reality to another. We are infinite souls. Those that have died or passed over, will be residing in another reality which exists in a different frequency from ours. We are beings of energy, we vibrate within a frequency range and so we experience everything within that particular range.

Beyond our physical body is what some refer to as the etheric body. This is the energetic body which surrounds us. When people invade our personal space they enter our energy body. Think back to when you were rooting out the frozen peas in the supermarket freezers, thoroughly engrossed in finding that last 1lb bag, somehow you sense someone is behind you. They have entered your energy field and subconsciously you became aware of it. Similarly we respond to the energy of others. Have you ever entered a room of strangers and thought crikey it's not very nice in here, or done the same thing and thought it feels lovely and calm in here. You are merely picking up the energetic state or vibrational frequency that exists in that place. Laws of physics state that like attracts like, and the same applies here. You are more likely to be attracted to someone with a similar energetic frequency as yourself.

Our energy body is alive and responds to how we are interacting with our environment in terms of our emotional state. When we are stressed or experiencing the negative emotions such as guilt, fear, sadness, hopelessness, depression etc., our energy field shrinks. Depressed people shrink within themselves, their energy is low and their field may only be a few centimetres away from their physical self. Contrast this with the person on top form, life couldn't get any better, their field will stretch outwards for up to twenty metres. I have read that students of yogis in India (these are enlightened beings of great wisdom and not some cartoon bear) often bathe in the loving aura of these illumined beings. Paramahansa Yogananda in his book *'Autobiography of a Yogi'* describes his experiences and training with modern-day saints and illumined masters of India, and further explains with scientific clarity the subtle but definite laws by which yogis perform miracles and attain self-mastery. It is well worth a read and will pass a few days if you are laid up as I was.

The energetic or etheric body can be seen by certain people who often quickly learn to keep such talents to themselves as it's deemed 'not normal'! All living things have these fields including plants and animals. The American military have even carried out extensive research into such things and can photograph the energy fields of individuals. As will be shown later in this part of the book, such knowledge is the foundation of Eastern approaches to healing. Chi, ki or prana is the universal life force energy which surrounds us and flows through us. Those who have watched the Star Wars™ films will be aware of The Force. This is where the concept of The

Force came from. This is not a new concept, such beliefs have been around for thousands of years.

I hope you are still with me at this point and have continued to read on just to see out of curiosity how far out I can really get. The good news is that this is my view without any illegal substances being involved! Nurse the medication is wearing off again....Next we come to the chakra system. Chakra is a Sanskrit word (one of the oldest languages on the planet) and it means 'wheel'. There are seven main chakras in the etheric or energy body with the first situated at the base of the spine with the seventh on the crown of the head. They are traditionally depicted in the form of a lotus flower and when this is combined with the symbolism associated with the wheel results in a circular shape spinning around its centre as individual petals unfold. 'So what are they for ?' I hear you cry. Chakras are present to enable that area of the body to have access to this life force I referred to earlier. The invisible etheric body where the chakras are located vibrates at a higher frequency than the dense lower-frequency physical body. In her book '*Healing Reiki*', Eleanor McKenzie states:

> "Imbalance can be seen in the chakra as either a slowing of the speed at which it spins and a diminution of its size, corresponding to underworking in the physical organs, or, conversely, the chakras can spin too fast and open too wide, also leading to physical and emotional problems. This is often experienced in the solar plexus chakra when the adrenals are overworked as a result of stress"

So you can see from these ancient belief systems which have underpinned healing systems for thousands of years that there is indeed more to us than meets the eye. It also highlights the link between our emotional state and our physical health.

As I mentioned in Part One I would re-visit the concept of transplants. We have over recent years marvelled at how we can now carry out transplants of organs. Heart transplants are now a routine operation and no longer make headline news as they did when the first transplant was made in 1967 by Dr Christiaan Barnard. Medical science has made tremendous leaps to reach the position today where transplants save the lives of many. However, there are numerous reports of the recipients of donor organs receiving more than they bargained for as they adopt personality traits of the donor. Gary Schwarz PhD, is Professor of Psychology, Medicine, Neurology and Surgery at the University of Arizona in the United States and has carried out research and details more than 70 case studies which validate the fact that consciousness lives on after we die. In one particular case, a young dancer received a heart-and-lung transplant. She had been an extremely health conscious person before the operation. The very first thing she did on leaving the hospital was to head for a Kentucky Fried Chicken outlet, and wolf down an order of chicken nuggets. This was something she would never have done before. Her personality was also observed to have changed. She became aggressive and impetuous whereas, before, she had been calm and conservative.

This girl decided to investigate what had happened to effect such a change within her. After much battling against medical bureaucracy, she discovered that her heart-lung donor was an 18-year-old man who had died in a motorcycle accident. His character was described by those who knew him closely as having been an aggressive and impetuous person who had a passion for Kentucky Fried Chicken (in fact, uneaten KFC nuggets had been found in his motorcycle jacket on the very day of his death). Medical science struggles to explain such phenomena, often blaming it on the drugs and anaesthetics. If you, like me, are aware that we are beings of energy then transference of energetic traits of the donor passing to the recipient makes perfect sense. It also highlights that we don't fully understand the process. For transplants to succeed on all levels for both the donor and recipient there needs to be input on an energetic level alongside the physical stuff. It is a dangerous state of affairs to assume that purely physically transplanting organs is all there is to it!

Next we come to the phenomenon that is the paranormal. The spooky world we are dared to think about. Have you ever met a medium ? No, but I've met plenty of large and the odd small, ho ho! A medium is merely a person with the ability to change frequencies and to tune into 'the other world'. Just as an aside, why is that when a Vicar hears voices it is God calling him but when it is Fred Bloggs from no 32 (who was always a bit odd and a bit of a loner as some neighbour who has seen Fred twice would comment) we call it Schizophrenia and pump them full of drugs ?

Dr Brian Weiss author of the international bestseller '*Many Lives Many Masters*' worked as a traditional psychotherapist. His young patient, Catherine was getting nowhere after eighteen months of traditional therapies. Dr Weiss turned to hypnosis as a last resort. He was both sceptical and astonished when Catherine began to recall past life traumas that seemed to hold the key to her recurring problems. Dr Weiss's scepticism was eroded, however, when she began to channel messages which contained remarkable revelations about his own family and dead son. Acting as a channel for information from highly evolved 'spirit entities', the Masters, Catherine revealed many of the secrets of life and death.

I was similarly sceptical back in 2003 when I went for a reading with a medium called Lorna who came highly recommended. Her first comment to me was that an old gentleman was present from 'spirit' and he wanted to thank me for helping him to pass over peacefully, particularly for reading his bible to him on his death bed, a fact known only to himself and me. I had nursed this gentleman and had indeed read his bible to him as he lay dying in a comatose state. My doubts quickly left me and I used the reading to help me on my spiritual journey with advice and guidance from 'the other side'. Much has come to pass that proves the information to be correct.

There are children in China that have become known as the 'Super Psychics', and these have been recognised and nurtured by their Government for the last 25 years. Schools and research centres are widespread throughout the country. By 1997, 100,000 of these Children had been recognised. Paul Dongo and Thomas Raffill in their book *'China's Super Psychics'*, state that one skill the children were able to develop was 'psychic writing', a technique where they were asked to imagine some written words on a blank piece of paper inside a closed pencil case. The case would be opened a short time later and on it were the words written in pencil. A girl from Shanghai called Xiao Kiong was the first to demonstrate this ability and so in 1981, researchers into 'Extra Human Functions' (EHF) at Yunnan Wenshan Teachers' College in Yunna Province selected 5 children with EHF for further training. It was soon found that when blindfolded, these children were able to see with their ears, nose, mouth, tongue, armpits, hands or feet. These tests were not right just some of the time, they were flawless. American new-age magazine *Omni* got involved when the tests were set up to check there could be no cheating. Interesting stuff !

There next comes the question then that if there is another realm where souls hang out is that what is called heaven ? Would it shock you to know that other dimensions exist. I have read that there are twelve dimensions. Even scientists at the forefront of quantum physics agree that in theory there could be such phenomena as multiple parallel universes and recognise through scientific research that there are more than the three dimensions originally thought to exist. We often think of ourselves as being supreme beings, masters of the Universe. Surely there cannot be any other intelligent life out there more advanced than us ? Wrong! As there are other universes and other dimensions so there have to be other life forms, other races, all part of that we call God. There are races out there that have the ability to navigate between dimensions through the use of inner technology, and by this I mean the ability to raise consciousness itself.

What do I mean by consciousness? By consciousness we mean our level of perception about ourselves and the world around us. The higher the perception, the greater the consciousness. Those who have had spiritual experiences have noted that their state of awareness, i.e. their consciousness, has been elevated beyond the norm, enabling them to experience existence from a whole new perspective. As our consciousness rises, then our psychic abilities will become apparent, which, for some will be quite an eye opener, possibly leading to a perceived increase in mental health problems until we begin to appreciate what is actually happening.

Spiritual researchers have looked into the ancient civilisations on earth of Atlantis and Lemuria and the fact that ancient Egyptian Mystery Schools developed knowledge and skills and through using sacred geometric principles were able to take initiates into a higher dimensional realm. The temples and pyramids we visit today were designed and built for this purpose. Human consciousness appears to be linked into a 26,000 year cycle known as the precession of the equinoxes. This cycle as I understand it relates to the slow wobble of the earth in an oval pattern. As Drunvalo Melchizedek states in his work known as '*The Ancient Secret of the Flower of Life*' as the movement takes us away from the centre of our galaxy so we fall asleep, losing consciousness in the process as we fall through the dimensional levels. As the movement begins to take us back towards the centre of the galaxy, we begin to awaken and it is possible to raise our consciousness at this time. The good news is that we are at such a stage where we are being given the opportunity to raise our consciousness collectively and build a better world for ourselves.

Now, make sure that your seatbelt is firmly in place, we are about to enter the world of quantum physics.....

A Paradigm Shift – The World of Quantum Physics

I am not going to reinvent the wheel here but aim to summarise what has been advocated over the past few decades by spiritual teachers who have studied health and how the world of quantum physics links into this. Do not worry, I failed O' level Physics (especially after nearly burning down the science lab after knocking over a lit Bunsen burner), so if I can understand it anyone can, trust me.

Dr Deepak Chopra, has written a large number of spiritual self help books including *Quantum Healing*, published way back in 1989. During his devotion to the subject of the relationship between mind, body and spirit with regard to health, Dr Chopra went on to envision a medical system based upon the premise that health is a lively state of balance and integration of body, mind and spirit. He is widely credited with melding modern theories of quantum physics with the timeless wisdom of ancient cultures.

What has happened over the past few years is that scientists carrying out experiments in the field of quantum physics discovered that particles of matter can behave differently when they are being observed under experimental conditions.

So what, I hear you cry? Well, that has massive implications for the spiritual community who have been saying for years that your thoughts create your reality. To sum it up, what we think can directly affect our world and science is now in a position to agree with this as the experiments carried out have demonstrated the link between thoughts and the behaviour of matter.

If you wish to expand your knowledge on quantum physics, and like me tend to struggle with such a concept, can I recommend a book to you entitled '*The Biology of Belief*' by Bruce Lipton PhD. Bruce is a former medical professor and research scientist whose work has looked in detail at how cells receive and process information. The information is presented in an easy to read style, even I grasped it first time! What he has discovered radically changes our understanding of life. We have been under the assumption in the past that genes and DNA control our biology from within the cell. In actual fact DNA is controlled from information **outside** the cell. This then proves scientifically that our thoughts (which are a form of energy) influence us at a cellular level, either positively or negatively according to what we think.

Now that has amazing repercussions on our everyday life. If what we think creates our reality that means that we are creating all those situations that appear to make us victims. In the third dimension where we reside at the moment, there is a delay in the time between our thoughts and their manifestation which gives us some safety margin in that we have time to correct our thoughts, especially where manifesting our fears is concerned. It is the old adage, "If you think you'll fail, you will" .

Our society encourages us to believe that we are not masters of our own destiny but that events just happen around us in some haphazard fashion, which is just not the case.

Why Are We Here?

Have you never wondered what it's all about? Why we are on this planet and experiencing this thing we call life? Philosophers gain PhD's out of such questions. I believe that we are all here to learn and to enable our soul to grow and develop. Some of us will use this incarnation to wipe out some of the karma we have carried forward from past lifetimes and hence help our souls develop along the spiritual path that we are all on. Karma as I understand it is the law of cause and effect and plays a central role in determining how life should be lived. Karma prevents us developing spiritually and is earned through our wrongdoings and misdemeanours. After all we have free will and being a human is not as easy as it looks! We choose incarnations based on what we need to experience to develop and thus can plan certain situations for ourselves to repay karma and to learn new things. Hence, "I must have been really wicked in a former life!" Have you ever wondered why the same situation keeps arising for you, it is perhaps, a lesson that you have not yet mastered. Good luck. I know I've had plenty. Other souls will have incarnated at this time to teach and be of service to others through these challenging times which paradoxically will offer us amazing opportunities to grow and develop. It's hard at times though!

Within us all there lies a piece of God, some wear theirs on their sleeve, some choose to keep their bit buried deep within never to get the light of day. No judgement, ultimately we are all part of the One. If you choose to hurt someone then ultimately you are hurting yourself. Call this loving force Mother/Father God, Source, The Creator, All That Is, The Universe, Great Spirit or The Divine, whatever label we give it it's there around us and within us.

As we exist in a physically dense dimension, the third dimension of twelve, life can be tough as we experience feeling separate from God and each other. Raising our consciousness in such a dense environment is not easy. The third dimension is classed as being one of duality, that is there is right and wrong, good and bad etc. Hence, the devil or evil has to exist for us to experience this phenomenon and have the contrast to good and the Light. Imagine the Star Wars™ films without Darth Vader, it just wouldn't work would it, just Luke and his mates playing football as there is no bad guy. During the 'peace and love' days of the 1960's many in the West experienced what love really is, unfortunately this was through being rocketed into higher dimensions through illegal drug use, notably LSD. The problem was then to re-create this feeling without drugs. We have lost that feeling of Oneness we had as spirits and have struggled to get that feeling and contact with love naturally. The good news is that we are heading towards a situation where we can regain that connection.

The Calendar Stops Here.....But It's Not The End of The World!

There is a great deal of information 'out there' in the public arena at this time which an ever increasing number of people are becoming aware of. I refer here to the subject of '2012'. One excellent book is simply titled '*2012 And Beyond*' by Diana Cooper and this gives an insight into potential changes that we may see over the coming decades, all from a positive viewpoint. If this comes to pass the world will be a truly amazing place to be and personally I'm glad I will still be around to enjoy it.

The majority of our indigenous tribes highlight this time to be of major significance in terms of human evolution. The Hopis predict that a period of purification and turmoil is the sign of the ending of their 4th Age and the beginning of the 5th Age which will be heralded by the appearance of a blue star from the heavens. Co-incidentally, comet Homes exploded in October 2007 to form a blue sphere visible to the naked eye! The Mayans call this period the "End of Time" and have prophesied events accurately in the latest five thousand year cycle with their amazing calendar. This calendar ends in 2012, however their most recent prophecy (in actual fact the first time they have spoken openly in the last five hundred years) states that incredible advances will be made by humanity during 'The End Time' which lasts from 2007 to 2015.

The Zulus believe that the whole world will be turned upside down. The Cherokee's ancient calendar ends in 2012. In Egypt, the stone calendar of the Great Pyramid also indicates that the present time cycle ends in guess when, yes you've got it, 2012! The Dogon tribe in Africa who are a primitive people have always described the star system of Sirius in detail and say that the "original visitors" will return in a spaceship that has the form of a blue star. The Incas refer to this time as the "Age of Meeting Ourselves Again". The Hindus write of this

Kali Yuga (a Yuga is an epoch or era) as the end of time and man and the coming Yuga as the age of many Enlightened Ones. The Maoris say that the veils will dissolve and there will be a merging of the physical and spiritual worlds. Add to this the renowned and highly accurate psychic Edgar Cayce (1877-1945) who predicted times of major change where we are now and the evidence is mounting that we are living in an unprecedented period in the history of humanity.

Now I don't know about you, but reflecting on the fact that all the ancient indigenous peoples on our planet along with an accurate psychic state that something big is happening right under our noses, then I start to think hang on a minute, there may be something in it.

Do not worry, though. There is nothing to fear, that is the last thing I want to create as it does the most damage in terms of us developing ourselves. We are the lucky souls that have been allowed to incarnate at this major transition for humanity. Why do you think that the population has risen so sharply over the past few years. We now have over six billion brothers and sisters on the planet. As I see it, it is inner technology that will see us through these times, and by that I mean developing ourselves in such a way to raise our energetic vibration and ultimately take the opportunities which will be presented to us to raise our consciousness. We have the opportunity to become enlightened advanced humans. Perhaps this is the first time you have encountered information such as this. The path forward you take from this point is entirely your choice. Personally I know that I want to stay around and take part in this monumental transformation.

Love – That Old Chestnut (Consciousness Is The Key)

Being a human being at the moment is quite a task. We are bombarded on a daily basis with a variety of media that challenges us. Take all the news programmes and newspapers giving us bad news and telling us what a bad world it is out there Then there are the advertisements telling us we must have x, y or z to be accepted by society. Conform or face ridicule is the underlying message. It is not easy to have all this thrown at you on a daily basis along with the unforeseen events such as the financial crisis and the global recession without it affecting you on some level. Usually this is to our detriment. We were not designed nor indeed were we ever supposed to experience such a catalogue of negative emotions. Fear and anxiety are the biggest culprits.

As an antidote to all this negativity we have that old chestnut called LOVE ! As Harold W. Becker puts it in his book *'Unconditional Love – An Unlimited Way of Being'*:

> "The greatest power known to man is that of unconditional love. Through the ages, mystics, sages, singers and poets have all expressed the ballad and call to love. As humans, we have searched endlessly for the experience of love through the outer senses. Great nations have come and gone under the guise of love for their people. Religions have flourished and perished while claiming the true path to love. We, the people of this planet, may have missed the simplicity of unconditional love. . .

Simply stated, unconditional love is an unlimited way of being. We are without any limit to our thoughts and feelings in life and can create any reality we choose to focus our attention upon. There are infinite imaginative possibilities when we allow the freedom to go beyond our perceived limits. If we can dream it, we can build it. Life, through unconditional love, is a wondrous adventure that excites the very core of our being and lights our path with delight."

Love is the answer but how do we get there then? Easier said than done though in these times in which we find ourselves. There are shelves full of self help books, workshops to attend, do this, do that, take this, take that... I've got the T-shirt, watched the DVD and taken every health potion known to man (a slight exaggeration but I think you get the picture), had healings of all kinds and yet here I am recovering from leukaemia. Without having had all the potions and healings I probably would be floating around in the spirit realm reviewing my life. Still the question remains, why did I experience leukaemia ?

Chapter Eight

Some Facts About Cancer

Incidences of Cancer

The word statistics tends to make people glaze over and switch off. For that reason I will try to keep the numbers to a minimum. It should also be pointed out that statistics can be used in a very manipulative way depending upon what you want to get across, as our politicians seem to do on a daily basis. That said however, you will gather from the previous chapter that I think that there is more than meets the eye as regards this cancer thing ! It is necessary in order to have an idea of how much cancer is a bane of modern society to look at how many people are affected by it. As Cancerbackup, the charity previously mentioned state on their website :

> "Each year more than a quarter of a million people are diagnosed with cancer in the UK, and **1 in 3** people will develop cancer during their lifetime. But cancer is not common in children or young people - it mainly occurs in the later years of life."

In the United States the figures make even more grim reading in that **1 in 2,** yes that's one out of every two people will develop cancer during their lifetime in the United States according to the American Cancer Society.

Looking back to the 1900's is interesting as cancer didn't appear to have the hold it has now. A Government research paper published in 1999, for example states that only 3% of deaths were attributed to cancer in 1880 compared to 43% in 1997. Critics would say that people would not have been diagnosed properly in those days. In addition there is the fact that the average age in 1880 was around 47 compared to 1997 where it had advanced some 30 years. So we live longer, it does not take away the fact that one in every three people is likely to develop cancer as we stand today. The future doesn't look too rosy either if you look at what the World Health Organisation (WHO) has to say :

> "As populations age in middle- and low-income countries over the next 25 years, deaths...from cancer will increase from 7.4 million to 11.8 million in 2030".

It also seems from what I have read that we in the developed West have twice the risk of being diagnosed with cancer than those people in the so called developing countries. This is not good news for our so called civilised society.

Pharmaceutical Companies: Friend or Foe ?

Make no bones about it, these companies exist to make money, and boy do they do it well. GlaxoSmithKline for example made a pre-tax profit of £7.78 billion yes that is billion in 2006 ! The recent swine flu debacle will probably lead to figures higher than this for the current years. Pfizer, the US pharmaceutical giant similarly reported net profits of $19.3 billion in 2006, up sharply from the $8.1 billion in 2005. In January 2007 they then announced 10,000 job cuts as part of a global cost cutting exercise! How much money do these people want to make. Morally I see it as being built on greed, others probably call that success. I could go on, it makes similar reading in terms of vast amounts of money being made by these organisations. Suffice to say that the pharmaceutical companies make a lot of dosh through us lot being ill. I have visions of Dr Severin Schwan, the Chief Executive of Roche Pharmaceuticals doing backflips and ordering champagne when he found out about the swine flu pandemic debacle. Roche are the company who are licensed to produce the antiviral drug Tamiflu, yes, that's the one that governments have been buying like we bought cabbage patch dolls back in the 1980's ! Have you still got yours ?

Iatrogenic illness is basically an illness resulting from medical treatment. A study into the concept of iatrogenic illness in 2003 by Gary Null et al somewhat shockingly found that in America iatrogenic illness is actually the leading cause of death in the United States. Even worse was the fact that prescription drugs were responsible for more than 300,000 deaths every year. The study went on to conclude:

> "US health care spending reached $1.6 trillion in 2003, representing 14% of the nation's gross national product. Considering this enormous expenditure, we should have the best medicine in the world. We should be preventing and reversing disease, and doing minimal harm. Careful and objective review, however, shows we are doing the opposite. Because of the extraordinarily narrow, technologically driven

context in which contemporary medicine examines the human condition, we are completely missing the larger picture"

Other studies have similar findings. A study published in The Journal of The American medical Association in 2000 by Barbara Starfield entitled '*Is US health really the best in the world*' found 225,000 deaths per year were down to iatrogenic events, concluding that this was probably an underestimate and that:

"If the higher estimates are used, the deaths due to iatrogenic causes would range from 230,000 to 284,000"

and went on to state that even the lower figure of 225,000 represented the third leading cause of death in the United States after heart disease and cancer. Given the similarity in health care delivery, it may be assumed that in the UK there is a similar picture in percentage terms.

So, what conclusion can we reach, are these providers of medicinal drugs friend or foe ? For me the chemotherapy I had saved my life so I have to think that without them I wouldn't be boring you rigid in such a wonderfully dry style. I will leave you with a hypothetical scenario though. As a background fact to this poser, a pharmaceutical company or anyone else for that matter currently cannot patent a natural product and therefore cannot make money from such things. So here we go. A scientist accidentally discovers that a type of grass when dried and taken as a herbal remedy has amazing curative powers particularly with regard to cancer cells. The cells transform back into healthy living cells within days. Would we find out about it and would it be adopted by our medical practitioners ?

Cancer Research

So, we have this thing called cancer which is threatening our society and indeed appears to be threatening our very existence given the fact that the incidence of cancer is on the increase at a rapid rate. What are we doing about it ? Well if you look at the Cancer Research UK website you will find that they are doing an amazing job of fundraising. Their annual Accounts for the year ended 31 March 2008 showed an income of £477 million with £420 million of that being raised by public supporters of the charity. Some figure that! Similarly in the United States, one of their charities The American Cancer Society had an income of $807 million in 2006-07. Cancer Research UK (CRUK) are proud to highlight that £333million of that money was utilised on cancer research in 2008.

Given these vast sums of money I am inclined to wonder whether the various charities which apportion such telephone numbers to research get value for money. What breakthroughs have there been ? Well, the Chief Executive in the 2008 Annual report states that :

> "Our ground breaking research is leading to new ways to prevent, diagnose and treat cancer, saving lives in the UK and throughout the world".

I would expect nothing else given the sums of money involved. Linus Pauling PhD, winner of the Nobel prize for chemistry and later another one for his peace work was considered to be one of the greatest chemists of the 20th Century. Speaking about cancer research he had this to say:-

> "Everyone should know that most cancer research is largely a fraud, and that the major cancer research organisations are derelict in their duties to the people who support them."

Strong words indeed from an eminent scientist, but given the lack of significant advances in eradicating cancer, it could be argued that this is probably justified.

Cancer research along with what now is a multi billion dollar industry appears to be entrenched in the *'targeted therapy'* approach. This can be traced back to the 1940's when two pharmacologists were recruited by the US government to experiment with mustard gas to investigate potential therapeutic applications of chemical warfare agents. In collaboration with a thoracic surgeon, they injected a related agent, mustine (the prototype nitrogen mustard anticancer chemotherapeutic), into a patient with non-Hodgkin's lymphoma. They observed a dramatic reduction in the patient's tumour masses. Although this effect lasted only a few weeks, this was the first step to the realization that cancer could be treated by pharmacological agents (Goodman *et al.* 1946). Since then it has to be acknowledged that there has been much research and development of more exotic chemotherapy treatments. The discovery that certain toxic chemicals administered in combination can cure certain cancers ranks as one of the greatest in modern medicine. Childhood acute lymphoblastic leukaemia, testicular cancer, and Hodgkin's disease, previously universally fatal, are now generally curable diseases. Nonetheless, cancer remains a major cause of illness and death, and conventional cytotoxic chemotherapy has proved unable to cure most cancers after they have metastasized (Wikepedia).

There are other branches of research such as gene therapy. The National Cancer Institute of America state the following:-

"Advances in understanding and manipulating genes have set the stage for scientists to alter a person's genetic material to fight or prevent disease. Gene therapy is an experimental treatment that involves introducing genetic material (DNA or RNA) into a person's cells to fight disease. Gene therapy is being studied in clinical trials (research studies with people) for many different types of cancer and for other diseases. It is not currently available outside a clinical trial. Researchers are studying several ways to treat cancer using gene therapy. Some approaches target healthy cells to enhance their ability to fight cancer. Other approaches target cancer cells, to destroy them or prevent their growth"

It would appear that this would come under the '*targeted therapy*' umbrella and although appears radical and potentially hopeful it still involves doing something 'to' the cancer patient as opposed to stimulating our own healing from within. I would add that with recent advances in quantum physics highlighting the fact that genes and DNA respond to stimuli from outside the cell and that according to Bruce Lipton "Only 5 per cent of cancer and cardiovascular patients can attribute the disease to heredity (Willett 2002)", this may be a bit of a red herring.

So what about the 'Alternative and Complementary' scene? Well certain therapies have had small trials conducted, often inconclusive and where they have shown a positive effect they have been dismissed due to the small numbers involved in the studies. All I would say as a non scientific type person is that conducting clinical trials costs money. A small group of therapists outside of the mainstream billion pound industry will probably find funding such trials nigh on impossible. Some studies have been carried out however. In October 2005 a report was published entitled '*The Role of Complementary and Alternative Medicine in the NHS*', commissioned by HRH the Prince of Wales. Its objective was to take 'a fresh and independent look – within a reasonable timescale – at the contribution which complementary therapies can potentially make to the delivery of healthcare in the UK.' It was produced by the economist Christopher Smallwood with the support of a consultancy team from FreshMinds, UK. Although not focusing on cancer which we are primarily interested in, the findings with regard to the whole issue of use of Complementary and Alternative Medicines (CAMS) in the NHS were interesting. Besides concluding that certain Complementary and Alternative therapies could be effective and, more, importantly these days, save the NHS money, the report commented on the research into CAMS as follows:

"Funds available for research into the cost effectiveness of CAM treatments should be increased. There is at present no paucity of financial support for CAM research which commands no ring-fenced government funding and only 0.08% of the NHS research budget and in 2003 accounted for 0.3% of the research budget of UK medical charities"

So there it is in black and white. A miniscule amount is spent on research outside what is accepted as the mainstream treatments that the conventional medical model has to offer us. CRUK highlight the perceived difficulties into research into the field of CAMS. Apart from the obvious lack of funding, these include a lack of time for medical doctors and complementary therapists to work together, difficulty in designing appropriate clinical trials and a lack of complementary therapists with research experience and knowledge. If we are serious about tackling cancer, given the billions of pounds invested in this industry each year, I would suggest that such problems could easily be overcome if the desire was there. From what I have read and observed though, another major hurdle for CAMS appears to be the fact that we tend to utilise them as a last resort and in terms of cancer treatments when the body has already suffered damage through chemotherapy, hence what trials have been carried out show those therapies in a poor light.

Searching for research into CAMS became a depressing affair. To bring a balanced view I decided that I needed to look at the organisations that are attached to and indeed formulating what care should be provided within the NHS. Organisations such as the Research Council for Complementary Medicine (which sounds grand but appears to have limited resources), NICE (The National Institute of Clinical Excellence) and NCRI (The National Cancer Research Institute).I have to admit to finding very limited success for CAMS with the majority of reports I found suggesting inconclusive evidence or the need for more research ! It seems a bit like the chicken and the egg scenario to a naive soul like me and that we are going round in circles and appear to be giving the matter lip service.

It is maybe at this point that I need to draw your attention to a little publicised report into the effectiveness of chemotherapy. In 1990, Dr Ulrich Abel, a highly respected German epidemiologist (a 'number cruncher' as he describes himself) conducted what has been to date the most comprehensive investigation of all major studies previously carried out on the effectiveness of chemotherapy. Dr Abel contacted 350 medical establishments to ask them for anything they had published on chemotherapy and also reviewed thousands of articles published in medical journals. He published his findings in the journal "*Biomedicine and Pharmacotherapy*" in 1992. So what did he find? I hear you cry. Well surprisingly he concluded that there was no scientific evidence available to show that chemotherapy can "extend in any appreciable way the lives of patients suffering from the most common organic cancers". I must point out that his conclusions were about certain types of cancer. As has been mentioned earlier certain others can be cured with chemotherapy. Even so why do we still sign up for chemotherapy on a daily basis in situations where evidence suggests it will do us no good ? For myself it was abject fear. I, like many others I am sure, did not wish to go against the power of the establishment that is the medical profession, which when we are in a very vulnerable position, often facing the guy with the scythe in the face, to then challenge what appears to be the consensus view is very difficult. What disappoints me is that we are not given a choice.

Cancer Treatment in The NHS & Elsewhere

As usual it would appear that we have followed America in terms of the accepted approach to cancer. America follows the 'consensus approach' to medicine. Medical consensus is basically a public statement made at a particular time on an aspect of medical knowledge and generally agreed by a panel of 'experts' as being the evidence based, current knowledge. In the UK, NICE the National Institute of Clinical Excellence develops clinical guidelines based upon the best available evidence on the appropriate treatment and care of people with specific diseases. Thus, we assume that we have a safe framework within which our healthcare is delivered, provided that this basic premise underpinning the whole thing is correct.

Generally speaking though, the current system treats symptoms. To give you a simple example, I have a headache, being conditioned into this system I pop in some paracetamol and the headache disappears. It could be that I was dehydrated which often results in a headache, a glass or two of water, I would argue would have served me better than the paracetamol, which like all pharmaceutical drugs, has side effects. We have become conditioned to focus on the symptoms and appear to have lost much of the wisdom that our ancestors possessed. General Practitioners have limited resources at their disposal, between 7-10 minutes for an appointment, this is a very short time for your doctor to get a whole grasp as to what is going on in your life besides the symptoms you present with. I have been fortunate in that my doctor will spend however long it takes to understand what is happening with me. He is always running late as a result but people find it well worth the wait. With budget restraints and targets to meet I wonder how long this will continue though.

Access to complementary and alternative medicine through the NHS appears to be somewhat of an ad hoc affair largely dependent on your postcode and luck. I have come across GP's who are also qualified homeopaths and acupuncturists and others who will refer people to such. Others see this as 'quackery'. In terms of cancer care, I was offered a weekly appointment for an aromatherapy massage or reflexology session. Where other treatments outside the mainstream are used it appears to be in order to aid the individual to cope with the conventional treatment, at least recognising that by increasing a sense of well-being in the person, they will be better placed to cope with the grim experience that is chemotherapy. It's a start I suppose and we have to be grateful for small mercies, allegedly...

Did you know that there are such things as NHS Homeopathic Hospitals in our country. I didn't until I came across one accidentally whilst searching for CAMS in the NHS. Well, it sounds exciting, there are homeopathic hospitals in London, Glasgow, Liverpool, Bristol and Tunbridge Wells. Quite how you get referred into one of these is beyond me, but I assume it will be through the more enlightened health professionals in those areas (the old postcode lottery scenario again) or through those professionals that have become so fed up of certain patients where nothing else conventionally has worked. Cynical, moi? As an interesting side note, did you know that the Royal family have always had homeopaths as their personal physicians from the days of Queen Victoria to the present. Coincidentally, they are also well known for their vitality and longevity!

The Department of Health's take on things is that the government acknowledges the increasing number of people who wish to take an active role in managing their health conditions and that CAMS are attractive to an increasing number of people. The DoH further states that CAMS could, in principle feature in a range of local services that local NHS organisations could provide, if they agree that it would be a clinically and cost effective use of resources and is in line with health priorities. Basically it's down to those who are in charge of your local health authority budget and whether they are open minded enough to consider CAMS as a cost effective resource. Primary care trusts often have specific policies on the extent to which their patients can be given access to CAMS. Within those policies, it is open to GPs to give access to specific therapies where they consider it in the interest of the individual patient. The cost-effectiveness, availability, and evidence in support of specific therapies are all issues that they take into account.

According to Andreas Moritz in his interesting book '*Cancer Is Not A Disease It's A Survival Mechanism*',

> "Many people who currently cannot afford costly medical expenses or medical insurance tend to seek more natural, inexpensive ways of dealing with illness; or else they don't seek any treatment at all. Given the high fatality rate among people receiving medical treatment, the risk of dying from no treatment at all is actually very slim."

Powerful words and he goes on to state that the concept of free healthcare as we have in this country encourages us to buy into this system. He cites the people of Cyprus who relied on ancient healing modalities until free healthcare arrived and then they adopted the modern healthcare system. It would be interesting to analyse the health of Cyprus' population now and compare it to pre-free healthcare.

I would argue that the concept of free healthcare for all is a superb model of care and we are very lucky to have such. I would have struggled to fund my treatment and may not be here now if it were not for the NHS. So, the basic ethos is correct in my view, however, it is the system that could perhaps do with an overhaul. I believe that all who enter the medical profession do so out of a desire to heal. Part of the original Hippocratic oath states:

"I will prescribe regimens for the good of my patients according to my ability and my judgment and never do harm to anyone."

Having said that, as we have already seen medical treatment or iatrogenic events were the leading cause of death in the United States, a not so well known fact. Medical student training is geared up to an outmoded Newtonian view of the physical world and ignores the discoveries of quantum physics, to our detriment. Medical students are trained in a system which discourages them to think for themselves particularly with regard to the underlying cause of disease. It is symptoms which are in the spotlight whilst causes appear to be ignored.

Maybe we have to look at the facts with regard to this system, remembering the fact that cancer now affects **1 in 3** in the UK and **1 in 2** in the US it would appear that this system no longer serves us as well as it could. I am not a researcher, but in attempting to gather statistics with regard to chemotherapy and survival rates I ended up giving it up as a bad job. The reasons for this decision came from the fact that as previously mentioned statistics can be misleading and can be manipulated to tell a different story according to whatever the compiler would have you believe.

In addition I have to mention that I have personal experience of the difficulties and complexities of designing clinical studies and then relying on the so called 'evidence'. Before undergoing my treatment for the leukaemia I was asked whether I would be prepared to be included in a clinical trial. This trial entitled, rather grandly, 'Medical Research Council AML15 Trial' (think we could jazz that up a bit) is taking place as I type in around 200 hospitals across the UK and basically is aimed at comparing different drugs against each other. Being a generally good egg and full of the 'aim to please' hormone I signed up. From then on my treatment was determined by a computer randomly choosing me a treatment protocol, I could opt out at any time and always sought the advice of my Consultant, Professor Jackson before proceeding. On reflection, however, certain things are ringing a few bells. The trial appears to rely solely on blood and bone marrow samples. I was never interviewed to find out if I was taking any other supplements or having any therapies which may impact on the results. I am thus a tad sceptical when people harp on about clinical evidence !

So, America and the UK share similar approaches to cancer, what about elsewhere in the world. I randomly picked a few other countries. China, for example, boasts as to having one of the most famous modernized cancer hospitals worldwide and offers treatments such as surgery, chemotherapy, radiotherapy, biological therapy, Intervenient therapy, and laser therapy in its major hospitals. I had obviously heard of the first three but what of biological, intervenient and laser therapies. The National Cancer Institute summarise biological therapies thus:

> "Biological therapy (sometimes called immunotherapy, biotherapy, or biological response modifier therapy) is a relatively new addition to the family of cancer treatments....... Biological therapies use the body's immune system, either directly or indirectly, to fight

cancer or to lessen the side effects that may be caused by some cancer treatments."

Intervenient therapy sounded exciting but turned out to be chemotherapy given directly into arteries near the cancer site, ouch! Laser therapy is the use of lasers to surgically remove cancer or pre-cancerous growths or to relieve symptoms of cancer. Often this approach will be used in those cancers on the surface of the body or the lining of internal organs. So, China with its history of Chinese medicine at least recognises the importance of the immune system in regard to cancer but also appears to have adopted the 'Western' model of treatment. Similarly, India, with its ancient system of Ayurveda, (a traditional system of medicine which is still practised throughout much of South Asia) sees the latter as a complementary approach and appears to have adopted a more Western approach.

All is not lost though, I then came to the jewel in the crown of the healthcare world, in my humble opinion that is! Germany!! Germany and Switzerland are the only countries I have come across that utilise Heilpraktikers as part of their healthcare system. A Heilpraktiker is the name given to a natural health professional in these countries (Wikepedia). To work as a Heilpraktiker (easy for you to say you should try typing it) does not require any formal qualification, but entrants to the profession have to undertake an examination and admission by the Public Health Office in those countries. There are approximately 20,000 Heilpraktikers in Germany offering a vast array of therapies. Bearing in mind that Germany was the country of birth of the father of homeopathy, that is Samuel Hahnemann, homeopathy also plays a major role in the healthcare system there. Homeopathy uses the concept "like cures like" as a fundamental healing principle. Hahnemann believed that by inducing a disease through the use of drugs, diluted many times from their original toxic state, the artificial symptoms induced would then empower the vital force of the individual to neutralise and expel the original disease. Around 20 per cent of Germans reportedly swear by homeopathic medication and there are about 6,000 physicians who specialise in it.

I then came across an advert for one of Europe's leading cancer centres St George's Hospital, located at Bad Abling at the foot of the Bavarian Alps half way between Munich and Salzburg. Here they offer what appears to be an essentially unique approach to cancer treatment in that they offer an *integrated approach.*

I quote from their website to give you a flavour of their ethos and what's on offer:

> "Integrative treatments combine conventional treatment modalities with complementary, non-toxic therapies to address the cause of disease.
>
> A fully accredited hospital with a staff of oncologists and other specialists, St. George's has superior diagnostic and treatment facilities. They offer an integrated approach to cancer care,

including nutrition, detoxification, homeopathy, acupuncture, phyto-therapy, Galvano therapy, mistletoe, vaccines and both traditional and complementary medicine."

If treatment addresses only the symptoms, the disease will reoccur because the cause of the disease has not been eliminated. Below you will find a list of integrative therapies offered at St. George's Hospital:

Classical oncological methods of therapy

- Chemotherapy
- Radiotherapy (in nearby clinics)
- Hormone Therapy
- Pain management

Complementary Treatment Modalities

- Hyperthermia (heat treatment)
  - Whole Body hyperthermia
  - Local-regional hyperthermia
  - Superficial hyperthermia
  - Interstitial hyperthermia (hot needle)
  - Prostrate hyperthermia (transurethral)

- Electrotherapy (ECT) or galvano therapy

- Photodynamic cancer therapy (PDT)

- Phototherapy (medicinal plants)
  - Mistletoe therapy, phyto nutrients, Chinese herbs

- Treatments with blood
  - Autohaemotherapy
  - Ozone-therapy, ozone-autohaemotherapy
  - Haematogenic oxidation-therapy (HOT)

- Treatments for pain
  - Acupuncture
  - Neural therapy (pinpoint injection of local analgesic)
  - Magnetic field therapy
  - Ultrasound treatment
  - Reflexology
  - Nerve stimulation
  - Drugs if needed
  - Permanent pain pump

- Biological Therapies
  - Immune stimulation with well-defined and effective drugs
  - Endogenous fever therapy with drugs such as interferon, interleukins   and bacterial derivatives
  - Active specific immune therapy ASI

(vaccine to activate self-defence)
- Dendritic vaccine
- Orthomolecular Medicine
- Vitamins, phyto nutrients, fatty acids, minerals, micro-nutrients, trace elements, amino acids and enzymes

- Homeopathy

- Detoxification

  - Hydro-colon therapy (intense intestine cleaning)
  - pH balancing
  - Far infrared Sauna
  - Direct current footbath (body check)

- Special Detoxification

  - Antioxidants (to detoxify from harmful metabolism waste products)
  - Radical scavengers (to neutralize harmful free radicals)
  - Intestinal ecology by probiotics
  - Special nutritional and fasting programs
  - Chelation therapy to eliminate toxins, carcinogens and heavy metals"

'Vorsprung durch technik' as they say in Germany! Wow! Some place to go for treatment. Now call me wildly deluded, but that to me sounds like a common sense approach to cancer treatment. It would appear to me that focusing solely on the symptoms of a disease does not make sense......it does make money though......

The Complementary & Alternative Scene

So why do I keep on referring to complementary and alternative medicine. Well it's not just me. According to the Smallwood Report expenditure on CAM in the UK is on a par with the United States. Latest figures from the National Health Statistics Report for 2007 show that in the US they spent $33.9 billion out-of-pocket on CAM products and services. Assuming the UK population is approximately one-sixth of that of the US this would suggest that for 2007 we in the UK spent approximately £3.4 billion on CAM products and services. This may be an under estimate given the fact that the Smallwood Report suggested that the market for CAM therapies "appears to be growing at a rate of 10-15% a year regardless of economic climate". It seems that as a nation we are increasingly seeking alternatives and treatments to either replace what the NHS system can offer or help us cope with it.

The other point worth noting is that when western medicine generally appears to treat these alternative treatments with derision and scorn, they are dismissing some healing modalities which are thousands of years old. Ayurveda, acupuncture and Traditional Chinese Medicine, for example date back to being over 5,000 years old. Many of these are based on principles which have been carried forward to more modern therapies such as Reflexology and Reiki to name but two. In my view he that dismisses such ancient traditions in the belief that modern man is somehow superior appears arrogant and his view is founded on ignorance. I would point out that ancient cultures appear to have enjoyed relatively better health than we modern types can claim today. Evidence to support such a statement is obviously limited, but there are instances of native American tribes such as the Navajo and Obijwa surviving smallpox epidemics introduced by white settlers through the use of herbal remedies. A tribe in the Himalayas known as the Hunza tribe were renowned for their longevity and lack of cancer until they became 'westernised', that is.

Nature provides us with a vast array of healing potential, we have tried to mimic these with limited effect with synthesised pharmaceutical drugs. What nature provides together with a knowledge of the spiritual and emotional body are vital components if we are to be truly serious about healing ourselves. Given the increasing numbers of individuals entering this arena it would appear that the tide is turning, especially given the fact that people are having to pay for such treatments themselves in 90% of cases (Thomas et al 2002).

Chapter Nine

What Causes Cancer (Why Me ?)

Introduction – A Warning......

This is quite a heavy and potentially overwhelming chapter where the tendency for us mere mortals is to probably switch off quite quickly and put the book in the latest charity bag. Please stick with it, what I am attempting to portray here is that in my view there are numerous *potential* causes for cancer. Ploughing through this chapter in one sitting can, therefore, be heavy going and leave one feeling that it's all very depressing and so I may as well do nothing. That is certainly one option and I do have to admit to losing the will to live by the time I got near to the end of it myself! However, if we are to rid ourselves of this terrible affliction that is cancer then we need to start taking responsibility for ourselves and begin to realise what is actually impacting on us on a daily basis. At least give yourself the knowledge to enable you to make whatever decision you do from an informed standpoint. Are you feeling brave ?

What is Cancer ?

The medical definition of cancer states that it is an abnormal growth of cells which tend to proliferate in an uncontrolled way and are able to invade other tissues. Cancer cells can spread (metastasize) to other parts of the body through the blood and lymph systems. Cancer is not just one disease but many diseases, with over 100 being medically classified. Most are named after the organ or type of cell in which they start. Breast cancer, colon cancer to give but two examples. The National Cancer Institute (a United States Organisation) state that cancer can be grouped into broader categories thus:-

- **Carcinoma** - cancer that begins in the skin or in tissues that line or cover internal organs.
- **Sarcoma** - cancer that begins in bone, cartilage, fat, muscle, blood vessels, or other connective or supportive tissue.
- **Leukaemia** - cancer that starts in blood-forming tissue such as the bone marrow and causes large numbers of abnormal blood cells to be produced and enter the blood.
- **Lymphoma and myeloma** - cancers that begin in the cells of the immune system.
- **Central nervous system cancers** - cancers that begin in the tissues of the brain and spinal cord.

The word cancer is the Latin for crab. We are all familiar with the star sign cancer the crab. Cancer was adopted to describe a malignancy, probably because of the crab-like tenacity a malignant tumour sometimes shows in grasping the tissues it invades. It is interesting to know and, indeed a medical fact that we all have cancerous cells within our body throughout our lives. Yes even you! Normally our immune system restricts the spread of such cells and the status quo is maintained.

So we have the medical definition out of the way, but what does cancer mean to the majority of us. I would suggest that fear is the response we have become conditioned to display. I was that soldier!! Apart from the basic survival mechanism the 'Fight or Flight Response' I would suggest that fear is basically a response we humans have to certain situations due to a lack of knowledge or understanding. In terms of cancer we only see it in the way that the industry portrays itself to us. We see misery, pain and suffering and the prospect of a visit from Mr G. Reaper with his scythe and black cloak. Putting the body under such emotional strain surely can only make things worse as the immune system will take a further battering from the stress associated with being diagnosed with 'The Big C'.

How we perceive cancer is obviously linked to our view of the world. If you look on our bubble of biology as being just that and nothing more then the medical definition will seem appropriate to you at this time. If, however you think that there might be more to us than just flesh and bone, and that there are the energetic and spiritual aspects to us then you, like me, may perceive it in a different light. For me personally as previously mentioned in Part One, leukaemia really has been a blessing for me, a real wake up call which has encouraged me to look at my physical, mental and spiritual life as a whole. I believe that aspects of these three were seriously out of balance to allow the leukaemia to develop. With hindsight it has been a gift which has enabled me to sort myself out on all levels and to truly heal myself and move on. Anecdotal evidence would suggest that the majority of cancer survivors talk of a major shift in their lives.

Are We Looking in the Right Place ?

If we believe that cancer is a purely physical disease, as our current healthcare system does, then we are right to plough millions of pounds into research looking into the various ways of knocking out cancer cells, be it through more costly drugs or gene therapy. There are however , as you will not be surprised to find out, other views as to the nature of cancer. *'Cancer is not a Disease, it's a Survival Mechanism'* according to Andreas Moritz. He purports that cancer is an attempt for the body to heal itself and argues quite convincingly that when cells are starved of oxygen often they are also existing in a toxic environment as changes have occurred within the body to prevent the elimination of waste products. Such cells, starved of oxygen and other vital nutrients, suffocating in their own waste, have a choice, either wither and die or try and survive through mutation into what are regarded as 'abnormal' cells. Hence it is the body's way of surviving, often when things are starting to get desperate. Genes also play a part by generating a new blueprint that enables the cells to survive without oxygen and even to be able to survive through utilising some of the metabolic waste products for energy. As Andreas states:

> "The drastic reduction or shutdown of vital nutrient supplies to the cells of an organ is not primarily a **consequence** of a cancerous tumour, but actually it's biggest **cause**"

This theory continues with suggesting that cancer only occurs where the channels of elimination and circulation have been consistently blocked for a long time. To get to the root of the problem is to look holistically at what causes such blockages. The sources may surprise you when you look at the host of risk factors that can impact on us detrimentally. To me this does make sense. What does not make sense is that if the human body is designed to survive and live it will somehow try to destroy itself as our current healthcare model would have us believe. As the medical establishment remain focused on treating symptoms and not root causes it would thus appear unlikely they would adopt such a theory even though it makes perfect sense to an ordinary humble person such as I. Whatever is going on what we do have to acknowledge is that the person who develops cancer is out of balance. What follows is a look at what, in my view, can **potentially** impact on us with a view to leading to cancer developing. Some of these I believe have been causative factors in my leukaemia even though professionals would dismiss many and stick to the 'there is no known cause' approach. I would say that I know my body and I have inner wisdom, as we all have. Somehow I just know !!

Lifestyle

We have a choice as to how we conduct our life, that is the great thing about free will. However, certain of these choices can become restricted in what we call our society. What do I mean by this ? What I am attempting to convey to you is the fact that we think we have free choice in all aspects of our life, but that free choice is very often dependent upon what 'the system' offers us. The 'system' I refer to here is based on what the government believe we need, what is good for us. Do you trust someone you've probably never met to tell you what is good for you ? Does our society provide everyone within it the ability to have a nutritious and adequate diet and minimise the risk factors associated with cancer ? Answer that yourself at the end of this chapter.

What follows is a look at those areas of our lives that I believe can impact on us negatively in terms of our health, particularly cancer. The last thing I want to instil upon you is fear. I am merely attempting to inform you about what is being said about potential causes of cancer. What you do with the information is entirely up to you. It is easy to feel overwhelmed and bombarded with information. All I would ask you to do is follow what feels right for you, use your intuition, I have found that the more often I rely on this the more I realise it is usually the right thing to do for me. I would add that it is better to make an informed decision having all the facts rather than one based on about 30% of the information available to you. If you are serious about this cancer thing, then it will result in some changes.

Finally in this section I have to mention the old favourites of smoking and alcohol, which are universally agreed as being linked to cancer. According to CRUK, the links between smoking and cancer are now very clear. Smoking is the single biggest cause of cancer in the world, and accounts for one in four UK cancer deaths. Tobacco smoke contains at least 80 different cancer-causing substances. When you inhale smoke, these chemicals enter your lungs and spread around the rest of your body. These chemicals, scientists have shown, can damage genes and important DNA. This can then lead onto cancer.

We were misinformed on this subject in the past, being told categorically in the 1950's and 1960's that there was definitely no link between smoking and cancer by those scientists who were providing health advice to those in government at that time. An interesting point. If it happened once, it can surely happen again on other matters.

There are theories regarding the link between alcohol and cancer, the strongest being that alcohol is converted into a chemical called Acetaldehyde. This is the chemical that causes hangovers but can also damage DNA and preventing it from being repaired, leading to cancer. Other theories are that alcohol increases the level of hormones such as oestrogen in the body. High levels could lead to breast cancer. Alcohol is also known to reduce the amount of folate in our blood, this is a B vitamin that our cells require to produce new DNA correctly and hence if this production is affected it could lead on to cancer. How you choose to use this and the information that follows is entirely up to you. Having explored all these factors, I discovered that they can make you feel like you are being bombarded with risks at every turn of life.

Stress - The Blight of Modern Living

It is widely acknowledged that we live in a stressful society, how this has crept up on us is perhaps a debate which could fill several chapters which I do not intend to examine here. Suffice to say that modern living exerts pressures upon us that our ancestors would find hard to believe let alone cope with. As humans, we come with an in-built system to respond to stress often referred to as the 'Fight or Flight Response'.

Basically this is preparing us to respond to a perceived threat and is readying the body physically to either fight this threat or to take the 'leg it out of there' type approach (I have usually found the latter works well for me!). Hormones such as adrenaline and cortisol are released which have a direct effect on us physically through speeding the heart rate and raising blood pressure, releasing glucose into the system to give us a burst of energy and strength and improving our mental sharpness. At the same time non-important functions such as digestion are slowed and we are encouraged to eliminate waste products to make ourselves lighter so we can run faster. A fantastic system don't you think. The body is truly amazing. A certain amount of stress is good for us, it makes us perform well in situations where we need to be on top form. However, this response was only designed to last for a short period of time. Modern living, I would suggest, means we are faced with prolonged exposure to situations we perceive as threats and hence the system is being used more than it should be.

According to The Stress Management Society,

> "The UK's government agency the Health and Safety Executive says there is a convincing link between stress and ill health. Its research with Personnel Today Magazine recently showed that over 105 million days are lost to stress each year– costing UK employers £1.24 billion. The research is based on responses from almost 700 senior HR practitioners and almost 2,000 employees."

The link between cancer and stress is more difficult to prove according to researchers. The American Psychological Association state that where animal studies have been carried out a case for a definite link between cancer development and stress has been made. However, research into this is a complex field and what is even harder is research with humans. The interactions of the many systems that affect cancer - from the immune system to the endocrine system - along with environmental factors that are impossible to control for, make sorting out the role of stress extremely difficult. A 1985 study by psychologist Janet Keicolt-Glaser, PhD, and her husband, virologist Ron Glaser, PhD, however, found that stress impedes cells' ability to repair DNA damage. Failure to repair DNA damage is one of the first stages of cancer development, many theories say. They have carried out numerous studies since then that highlight the fact that stress directly affects the body's ability to heal itself. There is a growing body of thought that our immune system is the key to the healing process, thus anything which inhibits our inbuilt defence mechanism from not functioning correctly surely cannot be good for us.

Furthermore, as Bruce Lipton points out in describing the biology of stress, it is the nervous system which invokes either a protective or growth response according to environmental triggers. When we are in protective mode, that is responding to perceived threats, we automatically inhibit the growth response and subsequently the creation of life sustaining energy. He goes on to say:

"The proportion of cells in a protection response depends on the severity of the perceived threats. You can survive while under stress from these threats but chronic inhibition of growth mechanisms severely compromises your vitality. It is also important to note that to fully experience your vitality it takes more than just getting rid of life's stressors. In a growth-protection continuum, eliminating the stressors only puts you at the neutral point in the range. *To fully thrive, we must not only eliminate the stressors but also actively seek joyful, loving, fulfilling lives that stimulate growth processes.*"

So there it is, the stress response is a necessary part of our biology, where it appears to initiate a chronic response in some individuals (and I include myself here), it does not serve us and can actually be detrimental to our health.

Food, Glorious Food....

One of the most important aspects of our health comes from what we fill our bodies with. Indeed, for me this is one of the great pleasures of life. Basically we are what we eat. (If you are feeling nauseous with the effects of chemo then I would advise you to skip this section and come back to it at a later date). So what is good for us? Almost on a weekly basis we have reports stating that this is good, that is bad, blah blah.... The Government recommends an intake of at least five portions of fruit or vegetables per person per day to help reduce the risk of some cancers, heart disease and many other chronic conditions. The Food Standards Agency recommend that:-

> "A healthy balanced diet contains a variety of foods including plenty of fruit and vegetables, plenty of starchy foods such as wholegrain bread, pasta and rice, some protein-rich foods such as meat, fish, eggs and lentils and some dairy foods. It should also be low in fat (especially saturated fat), salt and sugar".

The problem is that we are in the privileged position of having so much choice of foodstuffs. We want cheap food and thanks to intensive farming methods the industry has been able to deliver just that. In the 1930's, the average amount of the household budget spent on food was about 35 per cent. Nowadays that figure is less than 10 per cent. We appear to have moved more into buying convenience foods probably as a result of the pace of modern life which discourages spending time preparing and cooking fresh foodstuffs. There is the luxury of being in a position to buy prime cuts of meat which need little or no preparation whereas our grandparents would have bought less favourable cuts and utilised them by preparing them into tasty dishes.

I would suggest that if you are serious about getting your body healthy that you read Felicity Lawrence's excellent book *'Not On The Label'*. In this study of the British Food Industry Felicity discovered that there is more to modern food than meets the eye. After carrying out an in depth and usually undercover look at how certain food is produced she produced some horrifying truths about the food we eat. It is about being informed and giving our bodies the best chance of healing by ensuring that what goes into them is going to help optimise our healing ability. Certainly my diet has changed since all this cancer thing happened. Firstly though, let me take you on a brief whirlwind tour of our food industry to give you a flavour (pun intended) of what we are being offered.

Chicken – In February 2008 The Independent Newspaper ran a story stating that Tesco the Supermarket chain we all seem to love so much (just a hint of cynicism there) slashed the price of a chicken to £1-99. Amazing to think that for less than a couple of quid you get a whole chicken. What do you really get ? The low budget range of the poultry industry produces what are referred to as 'broilers'. The term refers to a combination of the two traditional methods of cooking: boiling and roasting. I will not dwell on the animal welfare side of an industry that has to produce birds at such a price where some farmers are making as little as 2p (yes that's pence) a bird. Suffice to say it's no wonder that methods have been utilised to increase growth rates. The lighting in the production sheds is on permanently to encourage maximum growth rates and many broilers are slaughtered after just six weeks, this after being given massive doses of antibiotics as a matter of routine to limit parasites and diseases. There is a European Union Directive due in 2010 which states that the maximum stocking density can be increased up to 42kg/m² provided certain token welfare issues are addressed such as better ventilation etc. This still gives the birds an area smaller than an A4 sheet of paper.

In processed chicken you are not always guaranteed to be eating chicken. Trading Standards officials have spent the last few decades battling against a multi billion pound industry. Tests on chicken nuggets showed that labelling was misleading and only actually contained 16 per cent meat (and chicken skin counts as meat!). There is a concept in the food industry known as MRM, or mechanically recovered meat. An excellent concept for a producer if you have lots of waste chicken carcasses on your hands. In this process the chicken carcass is pushed through machinery to provide a slurry containing protein. This pulp is then bound together with phosphates and gums. Another trick of the trade has been to add water to chicken to increase its weight along with pork and even beef waste, delightful. As Felicity Lawrence states:-

> "...it becomes clear that doctoring of our processed foods has not only become commonplace, it is also in many cases legal. Water is routinely added to catering chicken, together with additives to hold it in. If you've ever eaten a takeaway, a ready meal, or a sandwich containing chicken, the chances are that you will have consumed chicken adulterated like this."

Personally I want to know that what I think I am eating is exactly that and, to coin a phrase from an old Harry Enfield sketch hasn't been 'buggered abowt with'. Add to this the fact that however miniscule we are told they are, there are still residues of hormones and antibiotics within the meat, but more of this later.

Bread – It's not the bread 'wi' nowt taken out' that bothers me, it's all the stuff offered to us as bread that's full of things that never used to be found in one of our staple foodstuffs. When I was a lad, as the saying goes, bread was produced by local bakers, baked daily on the premises usually, bought and consumed within a day or two as it went off quickly. It tasted marvellous. Fortunately in our town we still have that rare phenomenon that is a local bakers which produces bread which transports me back to those heady days of my youth when men were men etc.. In the 1960's a major development occurred in the world of baking bread. The British Baking Industries Research Association at Chorleywood discovered a method of preparing dough for bread by submitting it to intense mechanical working, so that, together with the aid of agents to oxidise it, the need for the dough to be fermented for long periods was eliminated. This saved about 1½ - 2 hours in the baking process. It is known, not surprisingly as the Chorleywood Bread Process or CBP if you prefer the catchy version.

A major breakthrough if you want to bake vast quantities of the stuff. 80 per cent of our bread is produced this way. Unfortunately the process allows a much greater proportion of low-protein wheat. In addition the process also requires additives to make the process work correctly. For hundreds of years the baking of bread relied on four basic ingredients, namely flour, yeast, salt and water. Nowadays the modern loaf will generally contain hard fats which improves loaf volume and helps it to last longer. Thankfully there have been recent moves within the industry to reduce the use of hydrogenated fat which has been associated with heart disease. L-ascorbic acid (E300) can be added to flour as a treatment agent. This acts as an oxidant making the loaf rise more. Chlorine gas is used as a bleach to make white flour even whiter and is often used to substitute the natural ageing process of the flour. L-cysteine hydrochloride (E920) is used to make stretchier dough's. It may come from the feathers of ducks and chickens. Soya flour can be added as an improver to help bleach and assist with increasing the volume and softness of the bread. Emulsifiers are widely utilised to improve the size of the gas bubbles which in turn enables the dough to hold more gas and thus grow bigger whilst also helping with reducing the rate at which the bread goes stale. Preservatives are used to prolong shelf life. Use of controlled release microencapsulated sorbic acid is claimed to be a cost effective method of keeping bread fresh and mould free for up to two weeks according to UK company TasteTech.

Whatever happened to the good old loaf which tasted good and doesn't stick to the roof of your mouth as modern bread appears to. Have you ever tried having a conversation eating a modern bread sandwich ? You shouldn't be talking with your mouth full anyway! Sadly, only 3 per cent of UK bread is produced by independent bakeries. Fortunately we have one in our local town which, I fear will disappear if the plans for a new Tesco go ahead.

The Chorleywood Bread Process has coincided with an increase in the population of infections such as thrush which occurs because of a yeast organism candida albicans. There has been little research into this though. John Lister a master miller at Shipton Mill in Gloucestershire teamed up with his local allergy clinic to offer people claiming wheat allergies a selection of loaves fermented for different time periods. While allergic reactions remained with breads fermented for less than 10 hours as in the CBP, loaves fermented artisan-style for between 16 and 24 hours produced greatly reduced reactions or none at all. Gluten allergies seem to be on the increase, you can even buy gluten free battered whatever at our local chippy. Maybe this increase is just a coincidence!

Salad – This is good for us, we can now get access to salad all year round. Since 1992 it has even been washed and prepared ready to eat for us, lying on the supermarket shelves like little travel pillows. This Modified Atmosphere Packaging or guess what, MAP as the industry refers to it, increases the shelf life of salads by over 50 per cent. Normally this process involves lowering the oxygen content from 21 per cent to 3 per cent whilst raising the Carbon Dioxide levels correspondingly. Chlorine washes are used to disinfect out any bugs which may carry such nasties as E.coli. These washes are using chlorine twenty times stronger than a swimming pool! Unfortunately they also appear to affect the taste of the salad which is probably why we tend to smother them in dressings.

Research published in 2003 by The British Journal of Nutrition showed that MAP affects the nutritional value of the salad, most notably in the levels of antioxidants which are below the levels found in freshly picked salad. As Felicity Lawrence writes on the subject of chlorine washes:

> "Some chlorinated compounds are known to be cancer-causing, but there appears to be little research on those left on foods treated with high doses of chlorine, the process having evolved in an ad hoc way."

Pesticides – All perfectly legal and above board of course, as you would expect. The Food Standards Agency (FSA) inform us that pesticides are used for different reasons ranging from disease prevention to pest and weed control and preventing mould growth in transit and storage. "If pesticides were not used, this could affect the availability and prices of food" so state the FSA. It stands to reason that use of pesticides in food production will leave a certain amount of them on the food we eat. Indeed we are encouraged to peel our fruit, the problem is that as many nutritionists will acknowledge, the peel is often a rich source of antioxidants. Do not worry though, there is a programme under the eyes of 'The Pesticide Residue Committee' (PRC surprise surprise) which measures the levels on foodstuffs across the food range from this country and abroad. I wondered at this point if the PRC has a Christmas party and if so what sort of affair it would be and what would be on the menu ?

The Canadian Cancer Society highlight the fact that studies show there may be a risk of cancer through pesticide exposure but acknowledges that whilst the evidence is not yet conclusive, it is growing and certainly suggestive of this. What concerns me is the fact that whilst individual chemicals are deemed safe for use within the food industry, nobody seems to be examining how the human body copes with the chemical cocktail it may be exposed to on an almost daily basis. Good news is that the Cooperative group are leading the way through developing an industry leading policy to cover pesticide use on its produce, this has been updated recently to reflect the suspected impact of pesticides on the bee population. The latest statement on the subject is as follows:-

> "In line with our food ethical membership consultation, we have extended our banned and prohibited lists to 24 banned pesticides that will never be used on Co-op fresh produce and a prohibited list of 98 pesticides, that can only be used with a derogation."

At least there is a chink of light within the industry that maybe human health is becoming a priority over profit, in some quarters at least, let us hope this ethical stance is catching.

Antibiotics & Growth Hormones – Antibiotics can be used in farming in one of four ways. Firstly, to treat sick animals, secondly to protect healthy animals against the risk of infection, thirdly to protect an entire flock or herd on a routine basis against the diseases prevalent in intensive farming and finally, as a growth promoter to make the animals grow up to 10 per cent faster. In June 2007, a report by The Soil Association stated that a new strain of the superbug MRSA (short for Methicillin-Resistant Staphylococcus Aureus, thank god for abbreviations in this case) has been found in livestock continental Europe and this is transferring to humans. The report goes on to say:

> "Farm-animal MRSA is spreading on intensive farms in continental Europe. In the Netherlands it already affects 39% of pigs and almost 50% of pig farmers. In Dutch hospitals 25% of all MRSA cases are now caused by the farm-animal strain, and farmers are no longer permitted in general wards without prior screening. It has been found in chickens, dairy cows and calves and in 20% of pork, 21% of chicken and 3% of beef. It has also been found in farm animals and people in Germany and Denmark from which we import large quantities of pork."

In 2006 The Daily Mail newspaper ran a story highlighting the alarming evidence that beef raised with the use of growth hormones in the United States and Canada can trigger breast and other cancers . Despite the European Union banning the import of American beef which has been produced using a cocktail of hormones, John Verrall a pharmaceutical chemist and member of the Government advisory committee stated there are serious doubts over whether this ban is being enforced as there is currently no testing of imports for tell-tale hormone residue.

There is evidence of higher breast and prostate cancer rates in the US, where most consumers regularly eat beef from cattle injected with growth hormones. For example, the rate of breast cancer among women in the US is put at 97 per 100,000 as against 67 in Europe. Similarly the rate of prostate cancer in men is 96 in America and only 37 in Europe. Fortunately the European Union does not allow the use of hormones in cattle production and has prohibited the import of hormone-treated beef since 1988. The ban has been challenged by the US at the World Trade Organization and the debate is still raging between the US and the EU over its validity.

Genetically Modified Food, Godsend or Wolf in Sheepskin?
The fact is the world population is increasing on a daily basis, or so we are told. Indeed the global population is alleged to have doubled since the Second World War. With more mouths to feed there is little wonder that the food producers are under enormous pressure to produce more food for less. In response, statistical evidence provided by the International Food Policy Research Institute shows that production of food has tripled in global terms since the Second World War and since the 1960's has expanded mainly due to the introduction of crop rotation, the mass production and use of petroleum based fertilisers and chemical pesticides, expanded irrigation and the introduction of genetically superior cultivated crops. As previously emphasised we want cheap food and seem unwilling to spend more of our disposable income on food produced where less intensive methods are utilised. The use of genetically modified crops has sparked intense debate. Hailed as being the answer to supplying an increasing global population there are potential risks involved. Benefits are said to include:-

- GM crops are cheaper in the longer term

- Less use of chemicals due to in-built crop resistance
- Potentially better quality food

The other side of the debate tends to focus on the following:-

- Potential danger to the environment
- Potential risk to human health.

Bruce Lipton, an eminent research scientist states in his recent book '*The Biology of Belief*':

> "...tinkering with the genes of a tomato may not stop at that tomato but could alter the entire biosphere in ways that we cannot foresee.
>
> Already there is a study that shows that when humans digest genetically modified foods, the artificially created genes transfer into and alter the character of the beneficial bacteria in the intestine (Heritage 2004; Netherwood et al 2004)"

The potential risk to human health is difficult to assess as it is not known what long term exposure to such foodstuffs may have on human health. Most studies concentrate on the short term. There is very little information on this subject. Certainly within the farming livestock sector meat is being produced which is being fed on genetically modified foodstuffs. Currently within the European Union there is no legal requirement to label or identify meat that has been produced in this way. In the United States The Food and Drug Administration (FDA) are set to approve a genetically modified salmon. Produced by a company called Aqua Bounty this fish has been produced using genetic material from Chinook salmon and an eel-like species called the ocean-pout. This fish grows at twice the rate of wild and ordinary farmed salmon. Quite what impact this will have on human health only time will tell.

There is also a debate about Soya as a foodstuff. There are a lot of debates raging around the world when you start digging a bit! Labelled as the miracle food that would save the world from starvation, it is found in an enormous number of different food products. In Brazil and Argentina, the use of genetic engineering is increasingly being adopted in soya production, in the United States 80 per cent of soya grown is from genetically modified sources. In China, the soya bean has been grown and consumed for thousands of years. It was considered as one of the holy crops besides rice, wheat, barley and millet. Soya beans are versatile, and can be processed to produce soya milk, tofu, tempeh, soya sauce or miso.

Promoters of soya protein which, incidentally, was a by product of an industry established to produce soya oil, claim that it has health benefits which include cholesterol-lowering effects. In 1999 The FDA in the United States came out with a health claim stating that 25 grams of soy protein per day may reduce the risk of heart disease. Most soya foods are also low in saturated and trans fats, one reason why the American Heart Association has recognized soya foods' role in an overall heart-healthy diet. The FDA has also officially recognized recent research suggesting that soya may also lower the risk of prostate, colon and breast cancers as well as osteoporosis and other bone health problems, and alleviate hot flushes associated with the menopause. In 1998, The Advisory Committee on Novel Foods and Processes (part of the Food Standards Agency and probably another good organisation to be a fly on the wall at their Christmas party) responded to criticism from Greenpeace the environmental pressure group by stating that genetically modified soya was perfectly safe for human consumption. Soya is acknowledged as a complete protein rich in vitamins and minerals including folate and potassium. It can also be a good source of fibre.

Opponents of soya state that all the above is too good to be true but do acknowledge that organic fermented soya can be beneficial to health. Soya beans belong to the 'legume' family which includes other beans such as adzuki, red kidney and barlotti to give a few examples. Being a legume, soya beans traditionally have required fermenting to get rid of harmful components, traditional methods in Japan see fermentation for at least two summers or ideally 5-6 years before it becomes beneficial to the body. Modern production methods used to produce products, such as tofu, bean curd, all soya milks, soya infant formulae, soy protein powders and soy meat alternatives, such as soya sausages/veggie burgers use non-fermented soya. In this non-fermented state there are a number of potential concerns for health, namely:-

- Can contain phytoestrogens (isoflavones) which can suppress the thyroid and lower metabolic function. Soya can increase the growth rate of breast cancer cells. Soya can increases progesterone activity and more breast cell growth in menstruating women. Some researchers believe the rapid increase in liver and pancreatic cancer in Africa is due to the introduction of soya products there.

- Can inhibit protein absorption by blocking the action of Trypsin and certain enzymes
- Contains phytic acids which can block the uptake of essential minerals, like calcium, magnesium, copper, iron, and especially zinc in the intestinal tract
- Contains Haemaggluttin which can cause red blood cells to stick together inhibiting oxygen uptake and growth

So there you have it, a whirlwind guide to some aspects of our food industry. I was going to look into the ready meal industry but I am starting to lose the will to live, sitting here chewing on my organically grown celery stick, sipping my carrot juice! There is another important factor with regard to the food industry that I feel the need to mention, that of food additives. Much has been written on this topic and the detrimental effect on human health that additives such as aspartame (the well known sweetener that now appears to be in every soft drink on the planet – slight exaggeration here), can have. I believe it is important to be informed about what we eat. Whether you change your eating habits is purely down to yourself, but whatever you decide, do it from an informed standpoint. Follow whatever you feel is right for you, all I am attempting to show you is that as 'We are what we eat' then it is important to limit the amount of potentially damaging stressors on our body.

As an addendum to this section it is worth highlighting that an organisation exists by the name of The Codex Alimentarius Commission, sounds very important with the Latin bit. Formed in 1963 as a joint venture by the World Health Organisation allied with the Food and Agriculture Organisation of the United States with a remit to develop food standards, guidelines and related texts such as codes of practice under the joint FAO / WHO Food Standards Programme. The Commissions website goes on to say:

> "The main purposes of this Programme are protecting health of the consumers and ensuring fair trade practices in the food trade, and promoting coordination of all food standards work undertaken by international governmental and non-governmental organizations."

Sounds a good idea doesn't it. An organisation designed to look after the standards of food and make sure what we get is safe for us to eat. On 31st December 2009, the Codex Alimentarius Commission went global, and also links in to the World Trade Organisation. Countries not signed up to this organisation would find it very difficult to win any food related trade disputes. The United States, Canada, Europe, Japan, most of Asia and South America have been seen to sign agreements whereby their internal laws regarding food and drugs become harmonised to these international standards in the future.

As with all things, however, it would appear that there is another side to this story. There is a movement in the United States against what appears to be around the corner with regard to the control of our food. Rufina James in an article entitled '*The Sinister Truth Behind Operation Cure-All*' highlights some important points as to what we can expect under Codex if we allow it to happen:

- Dietary supplements could not be sold for preventive (prophylactic) or therapeutic use.
- Potencies would be limited to extremely low dosages. Only the drug companies and the big phytopharmaceutical companies would have the right to produce and sell the higher potency products (at inflated prices).
- Prescriptions would be required for anything above the extremely low doses allowed (such as 35 mg. on niacin).
- Common foods such as garlic and peppermint would be classified as drugs or a third category (neither food nor drugs) that only big pharmaceutical companies could regulate and sell. Any food with any therapeutic effect can be considered a drug, even benign everyday substances like water.
- Codex regulations for dietary supplements would become binding (escape clauses would be eliminated).
- All new dietary supplements would be banned unless they go through Codex testing and approval.
- Genetically altered food would be sold worldwide without labelling.

So, where in the past we had The Reformation (genocide by any other name at the instigation of the Church, nice one, peace and love etc) to get rid of those practising herbal medicine under the guise of a witch hunt, we now appear to have a more civilised approach that is Codex. Wave your herbalist goodbye if this gets the go ahead. I suppose at least they won't be burnt at the stake!

Another potential concern for us regards the Codex policy on food irradiation. Food irradiation is the process of exposing food to ionizing radiation to destroy microorganisms, bacteria, viruses, or insects that might be present in the food (Wikepedia). We could have a potential scenario where all foodstuffs are irradiated under the guise of eradicating potentially harmful substances. A 2003 report by Andrianna Natsoulas, entitled *'Codex Alimentarius and the International Politics of Food Irradiation'* appeared in the Public Citizen (Public Citizen is a national, not for profit consumer advocacy organization founded in 1971 to represent consumer interests). This report was published for the Toronto Food Policy Council. Excerpts show the dangers of widespread food irradiation thus:

> "The move to remove the upper dose limit ignores well-documented evidence that irradiated foods may not be safe for human consumption – including the formation of chemicals linked to cancer and birth defects........ The result [of irradiation] is a *radiolitic product,* never found in nature and linked to cancer and genetic modification. More than 40 years of scientific research has shown many health problems

in animals that ate irradiated food, including premature death, mutations, reproductive problems, fatal internal bleeding, destruction of immune systems and others. In addition, research has shown that *all* vitamins can suffer substantial losses due to irradiation. For example, 91 percent of vitamin B6 in irradiated beef stored for 15 months and 33 percent of vitamin B12 in meat can be lost due to irradiation.

This , along with potential increases in antibiotic and growth hormone usage in the livestock industry along with the re-introduction of previously banned pesticides should hopefully be getting us a bit edgy. Keep those eyes peeled.....

Emotion, Emotion, Emotion!

The link between our emotions and health is one which Western medicine tends to dismiss as being not proven scientifically. To examine the effect that emotions have on health and in particular the link to cancer is bound to be difficult due to the emotional rollercoaster that individuals experience *after* diagnosis. To get a true picture of the emotional state of people prior to diagnosis is obviously impossible unless we test every healthy person! Basically you have to use your own discernment again. I believe that part of my healing process has been to examine my emotional body, and that healing this has been a major part of my overall welfare. For other people this may not be the case. There is a theory 'out there' being developed by behavioural oncologists about the personality traits of those more prone to develop cancer. Known as the 'Type C' personality such traits can be summarised thus:-

- A tendency to deny and/or suppress emotions particularly anger
- Pathological 'niceness'
- An avoidance of conflict situations
- A need to be liked by others
- Harmonizing behaviour
- Over compliant to the demands of others
- High rationality
- A lack of emotional expression (bottling up feelings)

I read this and certainly ticked a few boxes when applying them to my good self.

Pan Mingji, in his book '*Cancer Treatment with Fu Zheng Pei Ben Principle*' states that Traditional Chinese Medicine (TCM) claims:

> "Rage harms the liver, excessive stimulation harms the heart, grief harms the spleen, great sorrow harms the lungs, and fear harms the kidneys. Though not necessarily precise, this belief definitely points out that emotional injury will affect the physiological functions of the qi (energy) , blood, viscera (organs), and channels, and lower the body resistance, resulting in disease. The human body is susceptible

to cancer when under emotional stress or disturbance. This is mentioned early in Chinese medical classics, such as *Yellow Emperor's Canon of Internal Medicine* and *Golden Mirror of Original Medicine*".

The belief is that the body should be in balance to be in harmony and to enable the qi (the energetic force that all living things need to sustain life) to flow naturally throughout the body. Changes to this harmonic state can occur through emotional changes, such as worry, fear, hesitation, anger, irritation, and nervousness. TCM views changes of spirit and sentiment as the seven emotions: pleasure, anger, grief, fear, yearning, sorrow, surprise. These are seen as the emotional and physiological reactions of an organism towards external changes in its environment. Emotional disturbance is thus seen as a reaction, this can be either excessive (excitation) or insufficient (inhibition) which will, if left unchecked, ultimately lead to disturbances in the flowing of qi and blood and the efficient functioning of the organs. If this situation persists, then illness is the result. Personally I think that such ancient writings and wisdom should not be lightly cast aside.

Deepak Chopra in his earlier work studied hundreds of case studies of instances where people had survived serious illness without the use of drugs or surgery. What he found was that in these instances individuals had gained access to a part of themselves he termed the 'infinite intelligence', that part of us that makes our hair grow, our heart beat etc. When accessing this, he postulated that they might have got access to what he called at that time 'phantom cell memory'. He suggested that inside malfunctioning cells was stored some old suppressed cell memories. These could be old traumas that the individual had suffered or old emotions that were buried and bottled up.

Science is beginning to make the link between emotions and illness. In a study published in The Journal of Biological Chemistry in May 2007,it was shown that the stress hormone epinephrine caused changes to prostrate and breast cancer cells in ways that made them resistant to cell death. "These data imply that emotional stress may contribute to the development of cancer and may also reduce the effectiveness of cancer treatments" said Dr George Kulik DVM, PhD, an assistant professor of cancer biology at the Wake Forest University in North Carolina, United States. Levels of epinephrine are sharply increased when we are exposed to stress and can remain high during periods of persistent stress or depression previous studies have found. So, not only may emotional stress trigger and continue the development of cancer, but it may well inhibit any treatments the individual undertakes if they are in a state of emotional stress. I will reiterate this last statement, a stressed patient may not benefit from the treatment being given. A system that ignores the psychological state of a stressed person being treated does so to the detriment of that individual. In addition to this there is much anecdotal evidence to suggest that illness can be linked to trauma and unexpressed emotions.

Geopathic Stress and The Wireless Age

Geopathic stress is something that the majority of us in Britain have never heard of. Certainly until I started to take an interest in what has the potential to affect my health I had never come across such a concept. So what is it ? Geopathic stress is the result of disturbance within the Earth's magnetic field. We are accustomed to living within the normal electromagnetic field of the Earth which exists as the Earth behaves as though it has a large magnet at its centre. The rotation of the Earth then creates electrical currents in the molten metals found within the core and this in turn is what produces the electromagnetic field. This is a natural phenomenon. However, problems can occur for us where this magnetic field is disturbed. This disturbance can be natural such as in the case of subterranean running waters, certain mineral concentrations, fault lines and underground cavities. Other disturbances can be man made as in the case of quarrying, mining, underground transport systems and through public utilities (sewage and water systems etc.).

Thousands of years ago, the sages of India wrote about the adverse effects of geopathic stress upon the human body. The impact of non-life supporting magnetic imbalances was initially recorded in the Vedas. In the West it has been Europe which has led the way with regard to this. In many European countries, having a survey for geopathic stress is a normal part of the process of buying a house. Geobiology or geoscience as it is known appears to be little recognised outside Europe. Indeed it was in Germany and Austria in the 1920's where the first crude discoveries were made linking geopathic stress with cancer and ill-health. The superbly named Baron Gustav

Freiherr Von Pohl was renowned for his skills in the field of dowsing, and in 1929 he was asked to dowse the small town of Vilsbiburg as at this time this town had the highest cancer rates in the whole of the region of Bavaria. He discovered a 100 per cent correlation between the beds of cancer victims and the paths of subterranean streams passing through the town. Further dowsing of the city of Stetten led to the city's medical scientific association acknowledging that the 'deadly Earth currents' ran beneath the beds of all the 5,348 people who had died from cancer during the previous 21 years!

It was George Lakhovsky that first used the term 'Geopathy' in the 1930's and then went on to suggest that geopathic stress in the human body can cause the body to vibrate at a higher frequency than normal and can have a detrimental effect on the immune system. He further suggested that people who sleep or work in geopathically stressed areas are thus more susceptible to viruses, bacteria, parasites and environmental pollution. Following this, throughout the 1940's up to the 1960's Ernst Haartmann MD studied cases and concluded that cancer was a disease of location. Austrian Otto Bergmann in the 1980's carried out 6,942 tests and found that geopathic stress can have an effect on blood pressure, circulation, heart beat and breathing amongst others. Englishman Ralf Gordon correlated cancers of the lung, breast and cervix during the 1980's finding that 90 per cent of those cases had geopathic stress. In 1985 Dr. Veronika Carstens, wife of former German Federal President Karl Carstens, published a study showing that there were 700 cases documented worldwide where patients with terminal cancer had regained their health without any conventional treatment after their sleeping area had been moved from a location where geopathic stress was evident to one in which there was no detectable geopathic stress. Dr Hans Nieper says in his marvellous book '*Revolution in Technology, Medicine and Society*' :

> "According to studies I have initiated, at least 92 per cent of all Cancer patients I have examined have remained for long periods of time, especially with respect to their sleeping place, in geopathically stressed zones."

This was from a man who treated many notable celebrities from all over the world including Ronald Reagan during his time as US President. In 1990 the United States Environmental Protection Agency stated:

> "In conclusion, after an examination of the available data over the past 15 years, there is evidence of a positive association of exposure to magnetic fields with certain site-specific cancer, namely leukaemia, cancer of the central nervous system, and to a lesser extent, lymphomas".

What exponents of this field of study state is that the geopathic stress does not cause the cancer itself but applies additional stresses to the body which lowers the immune system, opening up the pathway for chronic illness to occur. Certainly European medicine appears to take this matter far more seriously than we do in Britain and the US.

It would seem that the incredible advances in technology resulting in the majority of us using wireless devices means that our bodies now have to cope with increasing volumes of radio waves. The majority of studies so far have shown that there is no link to mobile phones and brain tumours, however, one recent study in 2008, carried out in Israel, where mobile phone use is high, researchers suggested that heavy mobile phone use (several hours a day) may be linked to an increased risk of cancer of the salivary gland. The latter it must be stressed is a very rare condition. Bearing in mind that mobile phones have been with us for quite a short period of time, what studies have taken place clearly cannot predict what effect long term mobile phone usage can have on health.

In 1993 a Dr George Carlo was hired by the mobile phone industry and certain American government agencies to investigate what risks there were to public health from mobile phone usage. He was given $28 million as a research grant. Much to the relief of those funding him his initial research after three years showed few problems with using mobile phones. Since then, however, Dr Carlo has continued with investigating risks and has now become vociferous of the fact that there could well be an epidemic of eye and brain cancers as a result of their use. In addition he has proposed a link between electromagnetic radiation and autism.

In addition to mobile phones there has been the recent increase in wireless computer devices. The Health Protection Agency states that electromagnetic field levels for WiFi equipment are much lower than mobile phones and :

"On the basis of current scientific information, exposures from Wi-Fi equipment satisfy international guidelines. There is no consistent evidence of health effects from RF (Radio Frequency) exposures below guideline levels and no reason why schools and others should not use Wi-Fi equipment."

There are a minority of vociferous opponents to microwave ovens who claim that they damage foodstuffs cooked in them or re-heated within them. This appears to stem from research carried out by Russian scientists who found that various vitamins such as the B complex, C and E vitamins (these are linked to the reduction of stress and the prevention of illness such as cancer and heart disease) along with certain trace minerals were virtually useless after exposure to microwave cooking even for a short duration. From what I have read the Russian government banned the use of microwaves in 1976, the ban being lifted after Perestroika. Evidence of this is difficult to obtain as you would imagine. All the statutory bodies overseeing our welfare deem microwaves to be perfectly safe. I suggest you do further research on this one and draw your own conclusions, we got rid of our microwave a few years ago, basically as we never really used it much and wanted the space for our radio! Smoking was harmless according to some!

Disease or Deficiency ?

There has been a theory around for a number of years that cancer is not a disease but merely a deficiency in the same way that scurvy was identified as a lack of vitamin C, being prevalent amongst sailors where access to fresh fruit and vegetables was limited. Adequate intake of vitamin C virtually wiped out this condition overnight. Having said that it was a number of years before the suggestion that vitamin C was the answer was widely accepted and utilised despite the evidence. If cancer is a chronic metabolic disease such as scurvy, rickets, pellagra and beriberi, then maybe a change in nutrition as in all these other diseases, it could be argued, is the way forward in preventing it.

Our modern lifestyle and diet has changed somewhat from our ancestors. Before any western influences indigenous tribes such as the Hopi, the Navajo , the Inuits, the Abkhazians and the Karakorum were all renowned for their longevity and remarkable health with a marked absence of degenerative disease. In particular, a remote Himalayan tribe known as the Hunza showed that they were long lived, often reaching over 100 years of age, with little or no illness and certainly no reported cases of cancer. In the early 1900's Sir Robert McCarrison, a brilliant English surgeon reported on the Hunza tribe as part of his study into the diseases common to the Asian people. In determining why the Hunza enjoyed such extraordinary health compared to their neighbouring tribes who lived in similar localities, the only difference he found was their diet.

The Hunzas practised a simplistic form of agriculture returning all organic matter to the land. They used no chemicals of any kind in their food production. Their food consisted mainly of raw fruits and vegetables with sprouted pulses, whole grains, nuts, milk products from goats and occasionally a small portion of meat, the latter usually on holidays or special occasions such as weddings etc. Chickens, due to their habit of pecking at seeds, were not kept due to the fact that seeds were like gold within the community! They would grow spinach, lettuce, carrots, peas, turnips, squash, young leaves and various herbs. Wheat, barley and buckwheat along with a large proportion of millet would make up their whole grains. This would be stone ground hence the whole grain would remain in the flour. They would eat nuts in the form of the Persian Walnut, almonds, pecans, hazlenuts and apricot kernels. The Hunzas grow fruits in the form of apples, pears, peaches , black and red cherries and apricots. It is reported that a man's wealth within the tribe is measured in terms of the number of apricot trees he has. Their diet would also include milk products in the form of raw unpasteurised milk, clarified butter (ghee), cottage cheese, yoghurt and sour milk. Fruit and vegetables are dried naturally in the sun for use over winter with no additives of any kind being utilised. Most foodstuffs are eaten in their raw state.

Apart from the lack of chocolate in this diet, it is interesting to know that it is high in vitamin B17 or Amygdalin. The latter occurs naturally in over 1200 species of plants around the world and used to be a regular part of our diet. However, since it tends to have a bitter taste, it has tended to be eliminated from our modern diet through selection and cross-breeding. Our consumption of barley, buckwheat and millet has given way to refined wheat. It is thought that this lack of B17 in our diet can leave us susceptible to cancer. The theory suggests that Amygdalin works alongside the immune system and attacks any cancer cells that the immune system cannot cope with. As the website www.anticancerinfo.co.uk states:

> "Amygdalin comes alongside the immune system and attacks the cancer cells directly. The cancer cells have within them an enzyme which unlocks the poison in the amygdalin, and in this way the cancer cells are destroyed. Normal, healthy cells do not have this enzyme. In fact they have a different enzyme which unlocks the amygdalin in a different way and releases nutrients and also a neutralising agent which would neutralise any of the poison it came into contact with. Researchers at Imperial College London have been experimenting using cyanide to kill cancer cells, and state that any poison that escaped into the bloodstream would be quickly neutralised by the liver."

In this sense it is marketed as more of a preventative approach than a cure as such. There are outlets selling apricot kernels which can be taken by those wishing to prevent cancer along with those who have cancer. Opponents of this approach argue that it is potentially harmful as apricot kernels contain cyanide as one of their constituent parts. For this reason the Food Standards Agency suggest a maximum intake of 1-2 apricot kernels per day. There is, as usual in all non-mainstream approaches, contradictory advice. The supporters of this theory suggest significantly higher doses than this. Certainly, anecdotal evidence is that the Hunza consumed well over

1-2 kernels per day and they lived to over 100! The charity Cancer Active give the following information about the action of vitamin B17:

"Cancer cells differ in a number of ways from normal cells. One difference is that the mitochondria, or power stations, do not use oxygen to produce energy, nor do they use the normal twenty something step process called the Krebs cycle. Rather they use only four steps and have a whole different energy production system and different set of helper chemicals (enzymes).In a cancer cell one of these enzymes, glucosidase, is present at 3000 times the level found in normal, healthy cells. Glucosidase has a unique action with B-17, breaking it down into hydrogen cyanide (which kills it) and benzaldehyde, (an analgesic). However, in normal cells where glucosidase is virtually non-existent, a completely different enzyme, rhodenase which is involved in the normal oxygen burning process, actually renders the B-17 harmless, converting it to thiocyanate, a substance which helps the body regulate blood pressure, and vitamin B-12. So, the proponents argue, B-17 is a seek and destroy missile."

Supporters of this approach suggest that the B17 molecule, if it is broken down in a certain way can produce cyanide, but as the enzyme to do this is only found in a cancer cell it is a controlled and safe release where it is required to do its job. Similarly, a synthesised form of the vitamin B12 known as cyano-cobalmine is known to contain cyanide which is involved in a large number of reactions with enzymes throughout the body, a deficiency of B12 is known to be linked to an increased cancer risk.

Cancer Active respond to the suggestions of possible cyanide poisoning thus:

> "Five kernels at any one time in a 90 minute period is the recommended maximum, and cancer treatments have to be properly supervised. Excess B-17 and cyanide byproducts have been known to build up in the liver. Each of us has different capacities and the cancer patient has an already impaired liver. A healthy liver has an enzyme, glucorinide that can detox the by-products, but in a cancer patient, this can be depleted. So, cyanide poisoning can result if excess is consumed. 1gm is the maximum recommended to be taken at any one time while the US Nutrition Almanac recommends a maximum of 35 seeds per day."

The emphasis has to be on the fact that as with any treatment or supplement it should be monitored by somebody who is competent and in whom you trust.

There is an actual therapy associated with this theory known as Metabolic Therapy. This utilises 'Laetrile' which is a concentrated form of Amygdalin extracted from apricot kernels in addition to a combination of special diets, enzymes, nutritional supplements and other measures designed to remove toxins from the body and to give the immune system a boost. Therapy also tends to engage the individual psychologically by promoting stress reduction strategies. The United States Food and Drug Administration have refused to sanction its use stating that as it is a synthesised product it needs to be authorised for use like any pharmaceutical drug, this has not been forthcoming thus far. At the time of writing such therapies are available within the UK and there are suppliers of apricot kernels. Research as you will no doubt guess is limited and does not satisfy the scientific and medical community. What research was carried out with regard to vitamin B17 was mainly done on patients with cancer, usually in fairly advanced forms. It would be interesting to carry out research on individuals who were taking this as a preventative measure. There are many reported incidences of individuals benefitting from using B17 and the National Cancer Institute of the United States noted in 1978 that 70,000 individuals had utilised this approach up to that point. There were and still are legal arguments taking place in the US about the use of B17 and laetrile.

Water Water Everywhere...

About two years ago I was washing up, that is a regular occurrence I might add, and on running the water I began to reminisce about my swimming days. The reason for being taken back in time was the smell emanating from the running water, it was as if I was in a public baths as there was a strong aroma of chlorine. This has continued ever since and resulted in us purchasing a water filter to make it taste like you weren't swallowing from the pool as I invariably used to when learning to swim. The World Health Organisation states that 2-3 mg/litre of chlorine should be added to water in order to gain a satisfactory disinfection and adequate concentration with a maximum amount for use of 5mg/litre. In the UK all public drinking water is disinfected before supply, this through the use of chlorine, chlorine dioxide or ozone and increasingly through the use of such methods as physical disinfectants such as ultraviolet light (Water UK). The European drinking water guideline 98/83/EC does not contain guidelines for chlorine. The water for our domestic use, we are told, falls well within WHO guidelines and is safe for us to use.

There are, however, concerns about the health impact of chlorine which incidentally appears to be the cheapest way to disinfect our water. These mainly concern the by-products known as 'chlorinated hydrocarbons' or trihalomethanes (THM's, try saying that after a glass of your favourite tipple or even worse with ill fitting dentures, stand well back....). Most THM's are formed in drinking water when chlorine reacts with naturally occurring organic materials such as decomposing plant remains or animal matter.

There is, however, an increasing body of evidence for an association between rectal, colon and bladder cancer and the consumption of chlorinated water. In May 1999 a report compiled by, wait for it.......The Committee on Carcinogenicity of Chemicals in Food, Consumer Products and the Environment (think I would bypass their Christmas party!) examined studies into the chlorination of water and the effect on public health. This report , passed to the Department of Health stated in its conclusions that:

> "It remains possible that there may be an association between chlorinated drinking water and cancer which is obscured by problems such as the difficulty of obtaining an adequate estimate of exposure to chlorination by-products, misclassification of source of drinking water (including the use of bottled water), failure to take adequate account of confounding factors (such as smoking status), and errors arising from non-participation of subjects. We therefore consider that efforts to minimise exposure to chlorination by-products remain appropriate, providing that they do not compromise the efficiency of disinfection of drinking-water."

Showering, bathing and swimming are also activities that can potentially carry a risk with regard to chlorine and other chemicals released into the atmosphere at this time. A study by Brown et al in 1984 published in the American Journal of Public Health (not my regular journal, I prefer The Beano™) concluded that skin absorption of contaminants in drinking water had been underestimated and that ingestion may not be the sole or primary route of exposure as had been thought previously. Certain studies have documented the presence in the drinking water of many potentially toxic volatile organic chemicals (VOC's). In having a long hot shower we may be getting more than we bargained for ! For someone like me who likes to come out looking like a prune, this is bad news!!

So, that is chlorine, what about the old fluoride in the water being good for you ploy? You will notice that up to this point I have tended to sit on the fence a bit, well ok a lot actually. Well I've just jumped off and boy does it feel good. Fluoride is a poison, fact. In the United States since April 1997 it has been law that all fluoride toothpastes have to carry a poison warning on the label. The warning cautions users thus:-

> **"WARNING: Keep out of reach of children under 6 years of age. If you accidentally swallow more than used for brushing, seek professional help or contact a poison control center immediately."**

The amount that is advocated as safe is pea size, how many adverts do we see for toothpaste with the whole brush full. In addition, there have been concerns over the amount of fluoride potentially being given to infants through baby formula being mixed with fluoridated water in areas where this is being done. Formulas are now being produced with low fluoride content.

If you are interested in reading the truth about fluoride I suggest you read Christopher Bryson's book '*The Fluoride Deception*'. The book highlights the fact that fluoride pollution was one of the biggest legal worries facing key industrial sectors within the United States during the cold war years. The publishers summarise the book as documenting "how a hitherto-secret group of corporate attorneys, known as the Fluorine Lawyers Committee, whose members included U.S. Steel, Alcoa, Kaiser Aluminum, and Reynolds Metals, commissioned research at the Kettering Laboratory at the University of Cincinnati to "provide ammunition" to those corporations who were then fighting a tidal wave of citizen claims for fluoride injury. The research was directed by Dr. Robert A. Kehoe, more famous for his lifetime defence of the safety of leaded gasoline (petrol). When the half million dollar medical study showed that fluoride poisoned lungs and lymph nodes in laboratory animals, the research was buried, until Bryson dug up a copy during research for his book. One leading scientist who reviewed the 40-year-old Kettering study suggested that its non-publication might have been responsible for an epidemic of emphysema among a key sector of the industrial workforce."

Fluoridation of the public water supply was basically a superb scheme to get rid of toxic waste from the aluminium industry, nice one. Apparently we had a law sneaked through in the UK in 2003 (Section 58 of the Water Act for those who like detail) which makes it perfectly legal for Health Authorities to demand water fluoridation within their area. This is being attempted in Hampshire where the South Central Strategic Health Authority has become the first to use this law by giving the go ahead for the Southern City Primary Care Trust to demand that Southern

Water add fluoride to the areas water supply probably from 2010 onwards. In the 3 month consultation period 72 per cent of the 10,000 local people questioned opposed the scheme. Despite this fact, in the name of democracy the Health Authority in their wisdom decided to still go ahead! At the time of writing the area is awaiting a judicial review due to the fact that the opinions of local people were clearly ignored.

There is a growing movement among the dental profession, particularly in America that is opposed to fluoridation through the water supply, suggesting that there is no benefit and that tooth decay is naturally in decline and that statistics are being manipulated to present a different picture than what is actually happening in reality. I have decided that if it is ever forced on us in this area I am disconnecting my water supply and digging a well! An easier solution, as well diggers are not to be found in The Yellow Pages is to fit filters which can get rid of chlorine and fluoride.

Vitamin D – Sunshine or Sunscreen ?

Vitamin D is a fat-soluble vitamin which acts in the same way as a hormone, regulating the formation of bone and the absorption of calcium and phosphorus from the intestine. It also helps in the movement of calcium between bone and blood and vice versa (The Vegan Society). Vitamin D can be found naturally in a small number of foods such as oily fish and eggs. Other fortified foods such as cereals have added sources. The majority of our vitamin D comes from sunlight on our skin. Sunlight triggers the formation of vitamin D in the skin, which can then be activated in the liver and kidneys for use within the body. Studies have linked a lack of vitamin D with depression, prostate cancer, breast cancer, osteoporosis and other degenerative disorders. A 2008 report published in the Clinical Journal of American Nephrology (not good breakfast reading material unless, of course you are a nephrologist) stated that the consequences of low levels of vitamin D "include increased risk of various chronic diseases, ranging from hypertension to diabetes to cancer."

The Food Standards Agency give the following advice in terms of intake:-

"Most people should be able to get all the vitamin D they need from their diet and by getting a little sun.

However, if you are pregnant or breastfeeding you should take 10 micrograms (0.01 mg) of vitamin D each day.

Older people should also consider taking 10 micrograms (0.01 mg) of vitamin D each day.

You might be particularly short of vitamin D, and so might want to think about taking 10 micrograms (0.01 mg) of vitamin D each day, if you:

☐ are of Asian origin
☐ always cover up all your skin when you're outside
☐ rarely get outdoors
☐ eat no meat or oily fish

Most people should be able to get the amount they need by eating a varied and balanced diet and by getting some sun. But if you decide to take vitamin D supplements it's a good idea not to take too much because this could be harmful.

Taking 25 micrograms (0.025 mg) or less of vitamin D supplements a day is unlikely to cause any harm."

Basically it's down to your good self to look at your diet and your sun exposure and decide whether you are getting adequate amounts of this vitally important vitamin. There has been much controversy in the medical world (just for a change) with regard to the amount of time to spend in the sun in order to get benefit from vitamin D production against the threat of skin cancer. Sensible advice appears to be to limit the exposure to sun and that sun beds are a definite no go area. France has banned the use of sun beds by those aged under 18. The consensus of opinion at the moment appears to be that 20 minutes exposure of the face and arms without sunscreen will generate enough vitamin D which is superior to that ingested through diet. It is important, however, to assess your skin type and check what exposure is safe for yourself as dark skinned people may need longer. The Australians appear to have a common sense approach to skin care advising to cover up by wearing a top, a hat and using sunscreen. As you will no doubt have gathered by now I am a bit funny about chemicals coming into contact with me. Cancer Active, the charity give what for me sounds like appropriate advice with regard to what we slap on ourselves thinking we are being healthy and sensible :

"Buy safe, toxin-free sun lotions, moisturisers and fake tans. Avoid those containing AHA5 (Alpha Hydroxy Acids) which exfoliate the skin's protective barrier along with damaged skin cells and PABA (para-aminobenzoic-acid) which causes irritation. Other baddies include propylene glycol, mineral oil, parabens, and skin suffocants bentonite, kaolin and lanolin, which can cause skin rashes. Research shows that chemical sunscreens mimic the effect of oestrogen.

The following list of chemicals is from a bottle of well known brand of Moisturising Sun Lotion we had in the house :- Butylene Glycol Dicaprylate/Dicaprate, C12-15 Alkyl Benzoate, Butyl Methoxydibenzoylmethane, Ethylhexyl Triazone, Titanium Dioxide, Bis-Ethylhexyloxyphenol Methoxyphenyl Triazine, Diethylhexyl Butamido Triazone and the list goes on......I guess you get the picture. Maybe putting your deck chair next to a petrochemical plant will have the same effect!

Garland et al in a 1992 study published in The American Journal of Public Health highlights the fact that in those countries where sunscreens have been recommended and adopted there has also been the greatest rise in skin cancer. "In the United States, Canada, Australia and the Scandinavian countries, melanoma rates have risen steeply in recent decades, with the greatest increase occurring after the introduction of sunscreens." Their conclusion to their study was that untested but wide-spread recommendations to the general public concerning the use of sunscreens with the aim of preventing skin cancer may actually be more harmful than advice to control sun exposure by more traditional means.

Ultraviolet (UV) light is generally divided into three sections, these divisions being made according to wavelength. UV-A (near UV) is what gives us a tan, UV-B (mid UV) stimulates the production of vitamin D whilst it is widely thought that UV-C (far UV) is the baddy that can lead to an increased risk of skin cancer. The majority of UV-C is blocked out by our ozone layer. Andreas Moritz in his book '*Cancer is not a Disease it's a Survival Mechanism*' lists these scientifically proven facts about ultraviolet light stating that it:-

- Improves electrocardiogram readings
- Lowers blood pressure and resting heart rate
- Improves cardiac output when needed (not contradictory to lower resting heart rate)
- Reduces cholesterol, if required
- Increases glycogen stores in the liver
- Balances blood sugar
- Enhances energy, endurance and muscular strength
- Improves the body's resistance to infections due to an increase of lymphocytes and phagocyte index (the average number of bacteria ingested per leukocyte in an individual's blood)
- Controls a gene that is responsible for producing a powerful broad-spectrum antibiotic throughout the body

- Enhances the oxygen-carrying capacity of the blood
- Increases sex hormones
- Improves resistance of the skin to infections
- Raises tolerance to stress and depression

Until the advent of penicillin, the preferred method for treating a wide variety of infectious diseases was through exposure to the sun and its ultraviolet light because this was so effective in stimulating the patient's own immune system. Niels Finsen received the Nobel Prize in 1903 for successfully treating skin lesions with tuberculosis sufferers through use of ultraviolet light.

With regard to sunglasses we again come to differences of opinion. Some advocate wearing them all the time in full sun. There are however those who advocate that ultra-violet has a beneficial role as indicated above and that exposure on the retina of the eye is beneficial and not harmful. Supporters of this belief would advocate not wearing sunglasses that block out ultraviolet light. Dr John Nash Ott started life as a banker but soon became interested in photography. As a by product of a subsequent career in cinematography he began to carry out important research into the effects of natural lighting on plants, animals and humans. Ott discovered that only a full spectrum of natural light (including natural amounts of infra-red and ultra-violet) worked to entirely promote full health in plants, animals and humans. In the 1980's and 90s, Ott also published a series of seven articles in the International Journal of Biosocial Research, a medical journal that studies links between physical and mental health. Titled '*Color and Light: Their Effects on Plants, Animals, and People*', the articles summed up Ott's decades of independent research, which was contrary to the established 'wisdom' of sunglasses manufacturers who warned of the "sudden" negative effects of full, natural sunlight on the human eyes and skin (Wikepedia).

In an interview published in 1991,Ott described experiments which showed that sunlight absorbed through the retina had the most dramatic effect on the pineal gland, this being of the greatest significance with regard to cancer. He stated that there were neurochemical channels from the retina to the pineal and pituitary glands, these being the master glands of the whole endocrine system that control the production and release of bodily hormones. This then regulates all bodily chemistry, growth and all organs of the body. Despite what we are led to believe about sunlight it would appear that certain studies have shown that cancers don't seem to survive for long in it. In one experiment, a tumour-susceptible strain of mice lived more than twice as long under full-spectrum light as they did under standard lighting, and rats exposed to full-spectrum light had significantly lessened tumour development. Six major medical centres confirmed these findings. Maybe the coolest dudes are those without shades or those with shades that don't block the beneficial spectrum!

Vaccinations

When we take responsibility for our health it is only natural that as part of that process we start to examine everything that we put into our body. Vaccinations should not be considered as an exception to this philosophy. How often though is it a case of visiting the local practice nurse or GP and being greeted with 'roll up your sleeve', the old 'slight scratch' ploy and away you toddle, full of what ? For those serious about what they have pumped into them I suggest looking on the Vaccination Awareness UK website (founded by Joanna Karpasea-Jones) or getting a copy of the book '*The Truth About Vaccines*' by Dr Richard Halvorsen, a GP in Central London who has some interesting facts after 5 years intensive research on the subject.

In the UK by the time our future generation is 13 months old, he or she will have been given 50 (yes that's fifty) vaccines (51 when they introduce the all new all singing all dancing all clucking chickenpox vaccine) ! I would imagine that as a new parent looking after a new baby it is a very vulnerable position to be in and with a massive heap of responsibility for the little person thrown in. It is easy to see how the pressure exerted on parents to immunise their offspring is so successful. At the moment vaccinations in the UK are purely on a voluntary basis, that said, however, it would appear that we are moving towards a scenario where the state has the right to overrule the parent's wishes for their children with regard to vaccination. Come in Mr Orwell and have a seat, now then about this book of yours....... So much for democracy. It is worth, at this juncture, to go back in history to the 1976 flu pandemic which wasn't. In the United States it was recognised that the vaccine given then was leading to a sudden increase in the potentially fatal neurological disorder called Guillain-Barre Syndrome. More people died in the United States from the vaccination than the actual flu – fact. The vaccine was withdrawn rather rapidly as a result.

Here I aim to save you having to go to the trouble of finding out what is in the more common of the vaccines that we are routinely given such as polio, the MMR (which has courted much publicity in its own right) and Hepatitis B. The cocktails include amongst other things:- Neomycin and penicillin (both antibiotics, so far so not too bad), human foetal cells, aluminium hydroxide, mercury, formaldehyde and aluminium hydrochloride to name but a few. What concerns me is that those giving these vaccinations appear to have no idea of what is actually in the syringe. Before you have any vaccination, it may be prudent just to ask what is in it and potential side effects. Since my last chemotherapy treatment I have been offered three vaccinations as I am clearly now firmly ensconced in the 'Vulnerable Persons' bracket as regards to my health. I have thus far refused vaccinations for influenza, pneumonia and swine flu. My immune system is compromised and I don't feel the need to bombard it with more things for it to deal with. It amazes me how efficient the health service has become with regard to vaccinations, but the cynical side of me realises that GP practices get paid for each arm they jab ! As with all things, make your choice from an informed standpoint, I would urge you not to just roll up your sleeve before finding out what is going into your body.

It's Those Free Radicals.....

Free radicals are basically atoms or molecules that have at least one unpaired electron. They are usually very reactive and unstable. I feel sorry for free radicals as they are given a really bad press. The consensus of opinion is that they are bad. They steal electrons from other molecules potentially damaging DNA in the process which as one theory goes, causes cancer. It is our interaction with our environment which potentially increases free radicals in our body. Exposure to pollutants such as cigarette smoke and chemicals are thought to increase free radical formation. In addition it is felt that the presence of toxic heavy metals in the body will increase free radical activity, multiplying it by several thousand times, possibly up to several million times. It does make sense to me to recognise that free radicals have been around as long as we have, so why are they suddenly being put in the dock and accused of being the cause of cancer ? Free radicals only seem to attack what already is weak and classed as potentially harmful to the body. So maybe it is a scenario that where the body's own lymphatic system can no longer cope with worn out cells and metabolic waste material that free radicals move in to help out, a sort of phase two response to survival (Moritz). Not in fact a primary cause but a response to an already ailing body.

Whatever role free radicals play, the role of antioxidants is widely agreed upon as being of immense benefit to our bodies. These are basically substances that prevent cell damage by free radicals. Antioxidants are the good guys, they seek out the free radicals and give them an electron, how kind. In the process they turn free radicals into waste by products which can then be eliminated by the body. In addition, these all round good fellows are able to repair damaged cells. So where can

I get hold of these chaps? The good news is that they are found naturally in fruit and vegetables. Good sources include yellow and orange vegetables such as sweet potatoes, carrots and pumpkins, green and leafy vegetables such as spinach, broccoli and fruits such as strawberries, kiwi and cranberries to name but a few.

Is There Anything Left To Worry About ?

Well I'm sorry to say that yes there is. I list a few of them below with a summary of the rationale for their inclusion alongside:-

- Heavy Metals – A study in 2007 by Mariea & Carlo published in the Australian Journal of Nutrition and Environmental Medicine (ACNEM, they would have to shorten that one to fit it on the cover!) showed a link between autism and the build up of heavy metals. Initiated due to the near sixty fold increase in autism since the 1970's with the most notable increase occurring in the last decade. The research suggested that electromagnetic radiation affected some individuals by reducing that individual's capacity for eliminating toxic heavy metals. Most emphasis is on mercury exposure through vaccines, dental fillings and through contaminated seafood. Where the body is unable to eliminate such substances for whatever reason, it is left vulnerable and with an increased risk of developing illnesses such as cancer. Raised levels of lead have been associated with such cancers as myeloma and leukaemia. Metals such as chromium and zinc have been associated with increased progression for a number of cancers (Moritz).

- Toiletries – Just have a look at the list of ingredients in your shampoo, deodorants, soap etc...... Enough said.

- Hair dye – Not that this is a problem if you have had chemo! If you intend to use them have a look at some of the chemicals contained in a number of dyes. Para-phenylenediamine and tetrahydro-6-nitroquinoxaline, both have shown to damage genetic material and cause cancer in animals. The European Union recently banned 22 chemicals from hair dye that failed to meet its safety standards but one chemical Para-phenylenediamine, is still used in the UK, despite being banned in Sweden, Germany, and France. Coal tar, a known carcinogen, is often used in hair colours. Formaldehyde is used as a preservative and has been linked to cancer.

- Air Pollution – In 2007 a research project by the London Breast Institute published its findings after setting out to determine whether living in an urban environment can impact on breast tissue. Breast tissue can be fatty, glandular or a mixture of both. Other studies have shown that women with breasts composed of 25 per cent or more denser tissue have five times the breast cancer of women with fattier breasts. The London study showed that women who lived and worked in and around Central London were found to have denser, more glandular breast tissue than those women who lived in more rural settings. It was hypothesised that such factors as stress and pollution could be significant in the findings where breast density is increased as a result of hormone disrupting toxins. Common sense dictates that air pollution is just another contaminant for the body to deal with.

• Bra's – Various studies have shown that pressure exerted on the breast through wearing a bra can increase the risk of breast cancer through impairing lymph drainage. It is also interesting to note that where indigenous peoples have become 'Westernised' and started to wear bra's, breast cancer rates have soared.

• Dehydration – The majority of us are probably dehydrated. The UK Food Standards Agency suggest an intake of 8 glasses of water a day. On average the body will lose between 1 to 1.5 litres of fluid a day. This figure obviously increases with exercise or in a hot climate. The cells within the body need to be adequately hydrated to maintain optimum health. The cells can run dry for a number of reasons such as regular use of diuretic beverages such as tea, coffee and alcohol, stress, and finally amongst others foodstuffs such as chocolate, sugar and artificial sweeteners. When cells become dehydrated it is thought that it could lead to a scenario that triggers the mutation process.

• Night Shift Work – The IARC (International Agency for Research on Cancer), a part of the World Health Organisation has classified night shift work as a possible carcinogen. Denmark has been the first country to pay government compensation to women who developed breast cancer after working night shifts for at least 20 to 30 years. Studies included in the survey by the agency included one published in the Journal of the National Cancer Institute which highlighted a 36 per cent greater risk of breast cancer in women who had worked night shifts for more than 30 years than in women who had never worked nights. It is known that shift work interferes with the normal circadian rhythms that we all have, our so called body clock. Interference of this function can suppress the immune system , reducing melatonin and damaging genes, subsequently leading to the production of abnormal cells. Us males are not ignored in these studies either as men who work night shifts are more likely to experience prostate cancer.

• Mammography is a specific type of imaging that uses a low-dose x-ray system to examine breasts. A mammography exam, called a mammogram, is currently used as an aid in the early detection and diagnosis of breast diseases in women. In the UK this involves three yearly screening of all women over the age of 50. Mammograms save lives, right? Sorry, they don't and that's official. A Canadian study of nearly 40,000 women concluded that "in women aged 50–59 years, the addition of annual mammography screening to physical examination has no impact on breast cancer mortality". The process can provide exposure to radiation approximately 1,000 times greater than that of an x-ray. It is widely accepted in the medical profession that the pre-menopausal breast is highly sensitive to radiation.

A form of breast cancer called ductal carcinoma in situ (DCIS) has been seen to increase by 328 per cent. This may be a coincidence...... Despite the fact that breast tissue is sensitive to pressure, mammograms involve considerable pressure being exerted on the breasts as they are compressed between the plates during the procedure which is acknowledged as being uncomfortable and painful. There is also a school of thought that if any cancerous cells exist prior to the mammogram, the procedure in itself could lead to the spreading of such cells. A study in 2000 by epidemiologists at the University of Toronto from large scale research found that monthly breast self-examination (BSE) following brief training along with an annual clinical breast examination (CBE) by a trained health care professional is at least as effective as a mammogram in detecting early tumours and carries no radiation risks.

In the UK the Breast Aware campaign suggests following the Five Point Code:

- Know what is normal *for you*
- Look and feel
- Know what changes to look for
- Report any changes *without delay*
- Attend for breast screening if aged
  50 or over

In addition the advice given with regard to changes to look for with regard to self examination is as follows:-

Appearance. Any change in the outline or shape of the breast, especially those caused by arm movements, or by lifting the breasts. Any puckering or dimpling of the skin.

Feelings. Discomfort or pain in one breast that is different from normal, particularly if new and persistent.

Lumps. Any lumps, thickening or bumpy areas in one breast or armpit which seem to be different from the same part of the other breast and armpit. This is very important if new.

Nipple change. Nipple discharge, new for you and not milky. Bleeding or moist reddish areas which don't heal easily. Any change in nipple position – pulled in or pointing differently. A nipple rash on or around the nipple.

There are other diagnostic methods available. Digital mammography, whilst still using radiation does so at a much lower dose. The x-ray film of the conventional mammogram is replaced with solid-state detectors that convert x-rays into electrical signals. These are then used to produce images that can be manipulated electronically. A physician can zoom in, magnify and optimise various parts of the breast tissue without having to take additional images. The extension of the NHS Breast Screening programme to women aged 47 which will be complete by 2012 will see the introduction of digital mammography for this age group.

The psychological effects of going through such a screening regime cannot be ignored. By actually having such a procedure draws the mind to the fact that there is a risk. I do believe that with the power that is within us, for certain individuals the fear inherent with focusing on cancer could well lead to the disease manifesting, a kind of self-fulfilling prophesy. In addition to this, Cancer Research UK states that about 5 per cent of women (about 1 in 20) who have a mammogram are called back, but "only 1 in 8 of these women will turn out to have cancer". So the other 7 "will be fine", apart from the emotional trauma and potential damage the increase in stress will cause to the body.

As with all information presented here, I would ask you to form your own opinion weighing up the potential risks involved with mammograms.

- Acrylamide – This is a chemical that is known to cause cancer in animals and is a probable human carcinogen. In April 2002 the Swedish National Food Authority reported the presence of elevated levels of acrylamide in certain types of food processed at high temperatures. It is unclear as to how it is formed, although highest concentrations were found in starchy food such as potato chips, French fries and bread. Acrylamide has been found in a range of cooked and heat-processed foods in other countries, including The Netherlands, Norway, Switzerland, the United Kingdom and the United States (WHO).It has even been found in home cooked food. It is not yet clear at what temperatures acrylamide is formed in food, but it has not been found in food cooked at below 120 degrees Celsius. So far it has not been seen in steamed or boiled food. Guidance on this matter is not very forthcoming due to the lack of understanding on the subject so far. Those involved in this are worried though. The Food Standards Agency advise cooking chips to a lighter colour and soaking them in water for 30 minutes before frying but ensuring they are dried before placing them in the oil. Other advice is to cook food at a lower temperature for longer whilst also ensuring that any potentially harmful bacteria are killed off. It has been a major concern at the World Health Organisation who are looking into gathering more research on the matter before putting out specific guidance.

It has been shown through research that cooking certain meats at high temperatures creates chemicals called heterocyclic amines (HCA's). These pose a potential cancer risk. Similarly nitrosamines are found in barbecued food where the flames have blackened and burnt meat and in particular the fat. Nitrosamines can cause cancers in a wide variety of animal species, a feature that suggests that they may also be carcinogenic in humans (Wikepedia). Studies have also suggested a link with bowel cancer.

A Spiritual Perspective - Mission Over, A Time for Change or Self-Infliction !

From a spiritual perspective, it may well be that the arrival of cancer, or any other illness for that matter, is a preordained event built into our soul contract before incarnation. It is my understanding that cancer may be taken on by an individual for a variety of reasons. The following list is by no means exhaustive:-

- o As part of individual or collective family karma.
- o As a method of exiting life which allows loved ones time to prepare for that individuals departure.
- o As a preordained method of leaving this life as agreed prior to incarnation – usually after completion

of events which allowed certain experiences and lessons to be learned.

○ As a wake up call and a spiritual kick up the backside to change and focus on whatever you were really meant to be doing as part of this incarnation. Look on it as a sort of safety net to ensure that your life purpose is adhered to.

○ As a warning alarm to alert you to begin to look after yourself

It is possible that in some cases individuals have such a negative belief about themselves that they create an environment at a cellular level where cancer is the result. It is as if the cells are totally fed up, so, they end up just giving up! As was mentioned earlier in the section on quantum physics, our thoughts influence us more than we realise, this can be negative or positive. When we become aware that this in indeed true, it then becomes imperative that we nurture ourselves and think highly of ourselves. Maybe in some circumstances where we clearly do not like ourselves, cancer is inevitable.

Past Life Baggage

Here I would like to refer back to the book by Dr Brian Weiss, *Many Lives, Many Masters*. As a trained psychiatrist, working as a prominent psychotherapist in his early career he states that he did not trust in anything that could not be proved through science. In 1980, a 27 year old patient called Catherine was referred to him seeking help for her anxiety, panic attacks and phobias. For the following 18 months Dr Weiss used conventional treatments to help Catherine overcome her problems. When nothing appeared to work he tried hypnosis which can often be used as a tool to help patients re-visit long forgotten traumas that have disrupted their lives.

In the following sessions, under hypnosis she regressed back to her childhood and brought out deeply repressed memories, namely swallowing water aged five when she was pushed into a swimming pool and being molested by her alcohol fuelled father when she was aged three. Catherine then went back further than this though into past life memories that appeared to be the cause of her recurring nightmares and anxiety symptoms. She remembered living 86 times in a physical body in different parts of the world sometimes as a male, sometimes as a female. Catherine was able to clearly recall the details of each birth, her name, family and physical appearance and the area in which she lived, finally recalling how she died in each incarnation. Through working out what issues she had carried forward from previous lifetimes, Dr Weiss was able to then work with her to eradicate these. All that Catherine told Dr Weiss about her past lives and, indeed about his own family was verified scientifically.

It might just be that we have brought with us into this incarnation energies that are detrimental to our health......

Wrap me in Cotton Wool !

So what is there left to avoid I hear you cry, as you gnaw on your organic celery and sip your organic freshly prepared carrot juice! Well, what I am saying in this chapter is that there are in fact, a whole host of potential reasons why cancer exists in our society. Some of these are, to me at least, common sense. Maybe it is when a number of these interact in an individual that cancer will strike. If you merely believe in the western medical approach to cancer then the following must make sense logically. If everyone has cancer cells within them, as is widely acknowledged, then why does it go on to manifest in some and not others. Surely it has to be to do with our immune response. An immune system struggling to cope with bombardment from numerous environmental factors as described will, inevitably, become overrun at some point. This is not rocket science (a good job given my accident prone past).

Other reasons, from a psychological or spiritual perspective may appear a little farfetched for some. It is easy to give up and ignore potential causes, after all with my leukaemia I am told that apart from radiation exposure the cause is unknown! Being a curious so and so I just had a feeling that there must be a reason why I was diagnosed with such a blessing. Wrapping yourself in cotton wool is a start, it means that you are beginning to look after yourself. There is a wise old saying

> 'If you always do what you've always done, you'll always get what you've always got'.

To me, cancer meant a time for change.

It is easy to look for blame as to why cancer exists. If you have cancer and want to apportion blame I would ask you please, not to blame yourself, this serves no-one, least of all yourself. Look at the system we reside in which for some currently creates scenarios where cancer is probably inevitable. We do, however, give our power away to that system. In researching material for this book along with my own experience I have discovered that one of the keys to personal healing comes from us taking responsibility for ourselves. For true healing to begin to take place it is necessary for us to look inwardly and not rely solely on external 'cures' although these, whatever we choose, undoubtedly play a crucial role. Part of this introspective examination is to realise that we are the masters of our own destiny. There are thousands of self help books around the globe which teach these principles, it took leukaemia for me however, to be able to effectively instigate the change required.

Why Me ???

I can imagine that by now all the budding armchair psychologists out there will be suggesting that the reason for this chapter is that I must have something to 'blame' for my cancer, that it is a part of the process following a serious illness to get mean and angry that it should have happened to me. On the contrary, I would advocate that this leukaemia thing has been the best thing that has happened to me. This chapter is merely to help to try and explain the potential factors that can cause cancer in the first place. I am not out to blame anything or anyone, indeed I would like to thank those factors that have allowed me to change my life in such a positive way. So, with that out of the way, let me share with you what I believe led to me experiencing leukaemia. (I would say to those that state that I cannot possibly know what caused it that it is my body, please do not patronise me and suggest that you know my body better than I do!).

To understand why cancer came to help me, for that is what it has done, we must look at where I was before it all happened. I was a quiet sort of person, I avoided conflict at all costs and would rarely challenge the views of others even if they were violently opposed to mine. Hence, I would rarely speak my own thoughts, my truth. I would present as a placid and calm person whilst under the surface there were often raging emotions such as fear and anger. I was not the most confident of people. Throughout life these emotions have been bottled up, stored somewhere out of the way. There was not much in the way of joy or happiness latterly in my life. There have been discussions as to whether a cancer personality type exists. There are several traits to this personality which certain factions believe leads to a greater risk of developing cancer. This was the old me, namely:-

- ○ Not coping well with stress
- ○ Highly conscientious, often responsible and caring (particularly for other people)
- ○ A desire to make others happy, often at the expense of their own thoughts and feelings (people pleasers)
- ○ A lack of closeness with one or both their parents
- ○ A tendency to harbour such toxic emotions as anger, resentment or hostility

Following on from this is the thought that deeply happy and contented people who live their life full of joy (yes there are such people on the planet who manage this without alcohol or drugs) rarely succumb to cancer. Maybe studies need to be carried out to look at how often cancer strikes after bereavement, redundancy, divorce and other life trauma. I suspect there will be a significant correlation.

So with my own character assassination complete, let us look at where I was in terms of life situation. I was working in a system which I didn't really agree with. There was a token lip service paid to holistic care, but the bottom line was that the healthcare system I worked in was the orthodox medical approach. To work within this system with a radically changing and different belief system could only lead to stress for me personally. As in the treatment of cancer by orthodox medicine I remain convinced that many people with mental health problems could have healing through other methods than drugs and psychological therapies which merely serve to paper over the cracks, again focusing on symptoms as opposed to causes.

So here is a summary as to why I believe Mr Leukaemia paid me a visit:-

- Suppressed emotions - a lifetime of aiming to please others and not speaking what I truly believed at the risk of upsetting others.
- Stress – caused through work and physically through over exerting my body which ultimately weakened my immune system.

- Geopathic Stress – I was sleeping in a bedroom with geopathic stress lines running right through the bed.
- A lack of joy and fun in life.
- Until the last few years, a lifetime of exposure to the usual pollutants, foodstuffs and childhood vaccinations
- Past Life Baggage – I have carried forward a vast amount of dense, negative energy from previous lives which led to my energetic field grinding to a halt.
- To give me a kick up the pants, to instigate personal change and to get on and do what I am here to do, fulfil my life purpose.
- To bring me closer to my loved ones and to potentially allow them to express their feelings which, in some, have long been hidden
- To give me experience of the chemo thing, the fear thing and all that a diagnosis of cancer holds in order to enable me to write this book, which ultimately I hope will help others
- To give me a different view of this world, showing me it is really full of loving and caring people. To have time to appreciate nature and take in the pleasures that each day brings.
- To basically give me a deep clean on all levels, after all you can't get much deeper than your bone marrow.
- To get me to look after myself in terms of mind, body and spirit, to gain confidence and to learn to love myself
- To learn to appreciate the mind body connection, in particular the link between emotions and the physical body.

This has been a marathon of a chapter and may well have helped you sleep on occasions! Whether you choose to make any changes as a result of reading this is entirely up to you. What I hope to have got across to you is the fact that causes of cancer are numerous and will differ from person to person. Until we begin to realise the fact that there are causes outside what is considered to be mainstream belief, then there will always be cancer within society. Where the issue of your own health is concerned within the current system, I would ask you to ask the question "Where is the money going?". The answer may well lead you on the path of wisdom. When we begin to take responsibility for ourselves and react accordingly, then there is the potential to eradicate this disease once and for all. May I wish you well on your journey through this thing called life and hope that at the very least this chapter has enabled you to make a truly informed choice.

Chapter Ten

Spontaneous Healings – What's That All About Then ?

Read All About It, Miracles Do Happen !

Such a phenomena does exist. Scientific types tend to get a bit hot under the collar when the phrase 'miraculous healing' is used, claiming that it camouflages ignorance as to what is actually taking place. That said, however, it is interesting to note that the Catholic Church has a committee based at Lourdes which examines spontaneous healings and then declares whether they are miracles or not. The spontaneous regression and remission from cancer was first defined by Everson and Cole in their 1966 book '*Spontaneous Regression of Cancer*' as

"The partial or complete disappearance of a malignant tumour in the absence of all treatment, or in the presence of therapy which is considered inadequate to exert significant influence on neoplastic disease."

The terms "spontaneous regression" and "spontaneous remission" are often used interchangeably. In medical literature, *spontaneous regression* tends to refer to the reduction of solid tumours, or neoplasms, whereas *spontaneous remission* is used when describing the reversal of a disease process that tends to be more systemic, such as leukaemia or lymphomas.

The scientific fraternity state that spontaneous remissions occur in about 1 in 100,000. I think that this is an underestimate due to under reporting. After all, a medical practitioner is hardly likely to make a song and dance about such things which buck the scientific trend and which cannot be explained within the orthodox medical approach. So why do spontaneous healings from cancer occur? Why is it that the likes of Cancer Research UK and other similar organisations around the globe are not investing some of their millions to look at what actually happens in these situations. Most orthodox cancer related websites do not even acknowledge that such instances actually occur. It is as if orthodox medicine dismisses them as not actually taking place, often using the old 'misdiagnosis ploy'! Is it a case, perhaps of the reasons for such remissions lying outside the belief systems of that orthodox medical approach which then has the arrogance to dismiss them as it cannot explain them?

Let us examine a few case studies of people who have had such healings.

- Brandon Bays – In 1992 this lady was diagnosed with a football sized tumour. Being from the 'Alternative Health' scene, she wanted time to try to heal herself as opposed to the surgery which the medical establishment wanted to perform immediately. She negotiated herself a period of a month. As it turned out it took six and a half weeks to be pronounced in perfect textbook health, this with no pharmaceutical drugs and no surgery. During this time Brandon nurtured herself through a healthy and detoxifying diet and sought the reason why she had this tumour. In doing this she found that in her case this was through a long since buried emotional trauma from her childhood. Her book '*The Journey*'™ describes in detail her story and also gives others a model to follow if they are in need of clearing buried emotions. This event changed Brandon and led her to share her findings to help others.

• In his book '*Perfect Health*' Deepak Chopra describes the case of a Swiss patient named Andreas Schmitt who was diagnosed with melanoma, a fast spreading and usually fatal form of skin cancer. After surgery to remove a growth on his back and removal of fourteen lymph nodes under his right armpit he decided to refuse radiotherapy. His doctors told him :

> 'Untreated metastatic melanoma patients may live only a few months; treated to the maximum, their life expectancy stretches out, sometimes by a few years, sometimes not. After five years, the number of long-term survivors is under 10 per cent. Within ten years, virtually no one is left alive".

Six months on from surgery a swollen lymph node appeared this time under his left armpit. Tests showed that it was   the return of the melanoma. He sought alternative treatment in America and met Dr Chopra. He was taught the specific Maharishi Ayurveda mental techniques that are taught to all severely ill patients in Dr Chopra's practice. In addition to this he undertook purification treatments to rid his body of impurities and he returned to Switzerland. Four months later tests showed no trace of melanoma in his body. Two years later the situation was the same.

- George was advised by his doctors to take care of his personal affairs after cancer returned in his second kidney, the first being removed due to cancerous growth some months earlier. George sought out the help of Andreas Moritz who, within three weeks, guided him to address the causes of his illness. Fifteen years later he is still enjoying perfect health.

- There are a number of medical case studies where spontaneous regressions have been examined. The majority tend to look at   each case purely from a medical perspective though, with only occasional daring forays into the world of psychology! '*Spontaneous Remission - An Annotated Bibliography*' compiled by Caryle Hirshberg and Brendan O'Reagan summarises a number of case studies and can be found at the website of The Institute of Noetic Sciences. I give here an example of the numerous case studies thus:

A 61-year-old man was found to have squamous cell carcinoma of the left hilum with metastasis to the left adrenal gland documented by needle aspiration. About two years later, the primary tumour is not detectable, and the adrenal gland is of normal size on follow-up computerized tomography. To our knowledge, this is the first documented case of spontaneous regression of squamous cell carcinoma of the lung with adrenal metastasis. "In conclusion", the author states, "Spontaneous regression of cancer seems to be a real phenomenon whose mechanism remains unknown. This area should continue to attract research, as it certainly harbours clues which may some day aid in further elucidating the mystery of cancer."

What Makes These People Special ?

I firmly believe that these people are no different to you and me. We are all special and unique. Spontaneous remission, regression or miracle cure, call it what you will, I believe that we all potentially have the ability with the right guidance and help to achieve this. So far there has not been a cancer that we know about that has not been survived by someone. This should give us amazing hope. What appears to take place here is down to a number of factors - not an exhaustive list by any means - which I will examine in turn.

Taking Responsibility - Crucially, it would appear that where such healings have occurred, the individuals involved have moved out of the 'victim' role that is currently so natural for us to adopt when diagnosed with cancer. After all, the health system we belong to tends to ignore causes of the disease and therefore leaves us no alternative but to be a victim. This thing called cancer just happened by some quirk of fate type scenario. In moving themselves out of this trap though, these individuals have taken the first step to taking responsibility for themselves. Often this is described as a change in outlook from being a dependent person to becoming autonomous, a master of one's own destiny. In working with whoever we trust to help us through situations such as cancer we become empowered by working in partnership and participating in discussions about our health and wellbeing and not being a passive observer who has treatment 'inflicted' on them.

Finding a Reason for Your Own Cancer – How can we begin to deal with something such as cancer when we are told in most cases that "We don't know what has caused it Mr Fee". In seconds we are turned into victims. Part of the process of empowering ourselves is to not accept this and to find out for ourselves what the cancer has come to tell us. If you were brave enough and managed to stay awake long enough to read Chapter 9, then you have a long list of potential causes as identified from a variety of scientific and spiritual sources. Do not be put off, this is not rocket science, in my previous existence as a psychiatric nurse I was never ceased to be amazed at how much insight us human types have about ourselves. Finding meaning in the cancer then allows for subsequently finding reasons to live.

Being Open to Change – The majority of cancer survivors will admit to being changed in some way after the cancer has left them. Again I state the wise old saying, 'If you always do what you've always done, you will always get what you always got'. This is basically suggesting that unless we make changes in our lives, the odds are that the cancer will return or not be healed. If I were to return to playing out exactly the same roles as I did previously, I am convinced that I would be inviting Mr Leukaemia back.

The system we currently subscribe to has a narrow view of the biological bubble that we spirits reside in. Until it moves away from this Newtonian view of the world and begins to recognise all the potential healing that is on offer through the world as seen by quantum physics, we will see ever increasing mortality rates through cancer and other diseases. We need to be the ones who take back our own power and become masters of our own bodies, making informed choices given all the scientific and spiritual knowledge available at this time. Where such spontaneous healings have occurred that have utilised methods away from mainstream orthodox medicine, I would surmise that a radical change in belief system has occurred within those individuals to encompass the quantum view that we are basically energetic beings whose thoughts and feelings have a direct impact on our physical body.

Optimism for the Future – Having faced the actual crisis of diagnosis and the pain and trauma that possibly follows (depending on what healings are sought), individuals reported discovering a renewed optimism for the future and a life that is meaningful and fulfilling. It would appear that dwelling on the cancer does not serve us, similarly fear is not healthy as has been demonstrated. The cancer can be seen as a challenge, with the person taking up the challenge and having a renewed desire and commitment to life. Experiencing joy, love and laughter as an inherent part of life can only be of benefit to us.

Strength and Fortitude - As we are all unique individuals we undoubtedly have different ways of finding that strength, but certainly an inner sense of wellbeing would appear to be a vital component of healing in these instances. This may come from a strong support network through a strong attachment to a significant other or an organisation which offers that support. A religious or spiritual belief and subsequent faith cannot be underestimated. Activities which can bring such states where stress is reduced and an inner peace is seen to include prayer, meditation and yoga amongst others.

Self Awareness - Individuals who have survived cancer have been observed to become comfortable within their own skin. This includes being able to express their own positive and negative emotions and feelings along with their needs, wants and desires, these from the physical, emotional and spiritual perspectives. They are able to say 'No' when it is required for their own wellbeing without experiencing the negative emotion of guilt which would be to their detriment. Entering this phase of life in a state of grace also appears to be of significance where allowing and accepting the situation are key factors along with supporting instead of the approaches of fighting and resisting we so often hear about. Knowledge and growth of the soul or spirit also appear to need to be considered.

Abandoning Fear – This is a major one folks. Whatever the fear may be, death and dying being common ones, fear does not serve us well and as has been shown can create illness and severely compromise the path to health. Those individuals who have passed through this fear state have given themselves a major boost on all levels, physically, mentally, emotionally and spiritually. How you choose to do this is up to you. There are shelves of books, DVD's and CD's on the subject.

Correcting the Imbalance – Where such healing has occurred it would appear that individuals have either consciously or unconsciously aimed at becoming an empowered and balanced human being living a life of joy. Rectifying the imbalance which caused the cancer in the first place is then a task taken on by the person where the majority, if not all the above factors are already employed to beneficial effect. Which healing modality is then utilised is down to the individual.

There are some potential scientific factors............

Infections – Although it does not appear to have been taken up in any great depth by the medical profession there is a long held view that infections can play a major role in the spontaneous regression of cancer. In 2005, a review of all literature regarding case studies of spontaneous regressions over the last 100 years by Hobohm was published in the British Journal of Cancer. This stated

"A large fraction of spontaneous regressions and remissions described in the literature was preceded by a hefty feverish infection. The hypothesis that fever can have therapeutic value can be brought in line both with successful historical attempts to apply fever using bacterial extracts and with immunological evidence. Putative beneficial effects of fever should as well act preventive, and indeed epidemiological studies show that a personal history of feverish infections reduces the likelihood to develop cancer later.......... Today we should be able to induce and control fever much better than 100 years ago. The discussion should be re-opened if and how to best scrutinise fever therapy in the future ."

Andreas Moritz similarly shares this view, going so far as to suggest that where infections are not life threatening due to an impoverished immune system, that the standard approach of suppressing infections is actually a medical malpractice and that lives could well be saved by allowing individuals to experience an infection which will potentially also rid the person of cancer as has happened in a number of spontaneous regressions as described.

Other Medical Type Bits Hinted at as Being Somehow, Maybe, Possibly, Fence Sittingly Linked!! – From a review of literature on spontaneous regression by Challis & Stam published in 1990 come the weird and wonderful sounding :

- ○ Apoptosis – "A form of cell death in which a programmed sequence of events leads to the elimination of cells without releasing harmful substances into the surrounding area. Apoptosis plays a crucial role in developing and maintaining health by eliminating old cells, unnecessary cells, and unhealthy cells." (MedicineNet)
- ○ Antiangiogenesis – This is where the growth of new blood vessels which feed a tumour is prevented.

And others include the straightforward such as:

- ○ Natural maturation of the cancer
- ○ Pregnancy
- ○ The withdrawal of the carcinogen
- ○ The endocrine system
- ○ Hormones
- ○ Post Operative Trauma

And finally we have to mention the good old conundrum that is the.....

Placebo Effect – This occurs when a patient receives a form of medication or treatment that has no recognised therapeutic value (a placebo) and the patient improves. The patient believes and indeed expects the treatment to work and therefore it does. This is the placebo effect and has been observed throughout medicine from psychological illness such as depression to physical symptoms such as arthritis of the knee. In a study by Moseley et al published in 2002 in the New England Journal of Medicine, a trial took place whereby three groups were given different types of knee surgery, one group receiving 'fake' surgery. The latter included the patient being given exactly the same pre- and post-operative care as those that had received differing procedures where actual surgery was carried out involving cleaning the knee joint out in different ways. The 'fake' surgery was to make three 1cm incisions in the knee area and the surgeon acted as if he was carrying out the procedure as normal but no instrument entered the knee at all. The results were somewhat shocking in that the placebo group improved as much as those who had received actual surgery! Members of the placebo group were later observed doing activities they had long since given up such as walking and playing basketball! The study concluded that:

> "In this controlled trial involving patients with osteoarthritis of the knee, the outcomes after arthroscopic lavage or arthroscopic débridement were no better than those after a placebo procedure."

Is there not the merest huge hint that there is a link between our belief and our physical body? Maybe this is just another area despairingly dismissed by orthodox medicine. Perhaps some of the millions invested in cancer research could be ploughed into discovering why this effect really exists, or would that save too much money, or even worse, he says cynically, lead to a cure.....

Personal Conclusions

Miracle cures, spontaneous regressions, spontaneous remissions, whatever label you choose to attach to this phenomena, there is no denying the fact that these do occur. It is sad that so few resources are being allocated to researching such phenomena, but this just feeds the argument that orthodox medicine is part of a billion pound industry which will collapse overnight when we take back control of our own destiny and learn to heal ourselves naturally. Even better would be eradicating the causes of disease in the first place.

This phenomena does, however, give us an insight into what is possible for each of us, potentially just around the corner. As our consciousness increases, so we awaken to different healing modalities as we discover our hidden potential. As Jesus said we will do these things and greater, when referring to his life including his healing. No doubt I will be accused of giving out false hope, but without hope dear friends we may as well pack up and go home now, last one please turn off the light....

Chapter Eleven

What Else Is There besides Chemo ?

The Eastern Philosophy

When you start to examine the healing modalities that originate from the East, it soon becomes apparent that the body is seen in terms of energy. Chi, ki, prana, ying and yang all describe energy. Disease or illness is seen as coming from a state of imbalance. As Deepak Chopra has said with regard to Maharishi Ayurveda (an increasingly popular system of holistic healing based on Ayurvedic principles which was started in 1980 by Maharishi Mahesh Yogi, who established an international network of doctors, clinics and schools dedicated to eliminating disease):

> "Our goal is to reach the level of perfect balance
> that lies within every patient, no matter how sick.
> Experiencing this level brings healing, in and of
> itself, using the body's own methods".

Ayurvedic medicine or Ayurveda as it is also called is one of the world's oldest healing systems which originated in India. The term Ayurveda combines the Sanskrit words *ayur* (life) and *veda* (science or knowledge). Thus, Ayurveda means 'the science of life'. Its aim is to integrate and balance the body, mind and spirit, using a variety of natural products and techniques aimed at cleansing the body in order to restore balance. Approximately 80 per cent of the Indian population use this either exclusively or combined with Western medicine.

Traditional Chinese Medicine or TCM, as it is also jazzily known, has a history over 3,000 years old. It has formed a unique system to diagnose and cure illness and encompasses therapies such as acupuncture, herbal medicine along with qigong exercises and massage. All are aimed at bringing the body back to a balanced and subsequently healthy state. It is founded on the principles of yin and yang along with the Five Elements theory. Yin and Yang represent the forces of duality that exist at this time. Good and bad, above and below, day and night, and extends into our emotional states, without experiencing pain we would not know joy. It is natural for us to fluctuate between yin and yang throughout our normal daily routines, however, where the balance is consistently altered and one (either yin or yang) is seen to dominate the other then illness and disease is seen to occur. The Five Elements theory follows Chinese philosophy which recognises five distinct elements of cyclical change, namely, water, wood, fire, earth and metal. These elements can be related to the four seasons and also relate to different colours, emotions, taste and various organs of the body, and are seen in the context of processes of energy manifestation.

So, we have looked at just two Eastern systems based on the body being a balanced energy system and recognising that when this goes awry then illness and disease follow. Thanks to quantum physics it is now possible to link such concepts as qi,chi or prana to science. The concept of this universal energy field (The Force of the Star Wars™ films as previously mentioned) is now called the Quantum Field in scientific circles. Einstein with his E=mc² basically is saying that energy and matter are one. As American physicist, Barbara Brennan, states in her book 'The Hands of Light':

> "Through experiments over the past few decades physicists have discovered matter to be completely mutable into other particles or energy and vice-versa and on a subatomic level, matter does not exist with certainty in definite places, but rather shows 'tendencies' to exist. Quantum physics is beginning to realise that the Universe appears to be a dynamic web of interconnected and inseparable energy patterns. If the universe is indeed composed of such a web, there is logically no such thing as a part. This implies we are not separated parts of a whole but rather we are the Whole."

We appear to be at a major crossroads where science and spirituality are merging. What impact this will have on the health services of the future only time will tell.

My Story

I have touched on therapies besides chemotherapy that I have utilised in Part One of the book. Here I will go into a bit more detail to give you an insight into what the therapies I used are about and to demonstrate how skilled the practitioners are that I have been privileged to have met. All have played a part along my journey to where I am at this point and have contributed to the profound changes that have taken place in my life. Reflecting back I can see that things happened exactly as they were meant to, I am exactly where I am supposed to be at this moment. I have experienced what I have up to this point for a reason, perhaps that reason is so that I can impart this information to the likes of yourselves and help others through the difficult periods that cancer currently, inevitably brings.

Back in 2001 was when it all really started. I was, with hindsight, probably on the edge of some sort of breakdown. Working in the field of mental health I knew that pills of some sort would be the answer if I went to see my GP. At that time I was looking into alternatives and had read about Reiki. Coincidentally, one of our neighbours had been to see a Reiki practitioner who lived about 7 or 8 miles away and thoroughly recommended it. I booked an appointment and had a wonderful healing experience, I floated out afterwards totally calm without a care in the world. Something in me awoke at that time, life has never really been the same since. I was so impressed that I didn't buy the company but instead trained how to be a practitioner myself. I began to use it as a part of my nursing practice. Gradually though I was slipping back into the caring for everyone else but me!

A couple of years later Sandra and I attended a Flower of Life Workshop run by an amazing person by the name of Anne Ward (Anne still laughs now when we explain that we chose her because she sounded the most 'normal', a lot of the other facilitators sounded strange and had somewhat bizarre names!). This workshop teaches amongst other things the concepts of the Merkaba meditation, sacred geometry and methods to integrate the left brain (the mind) and the right brain (heart/feeling/intuition). For those inquisitive souls amongst you, more information is available at www.floweroflife.org. I am telling you this because Anne is also an exceptional healer, working with energy and with sound, aiming to release dense and painful energies and thus facilitate healing and growth.

From 2006 onwards I sought out the help of Anne, who was giving me healings as I felt I needed them. This would mean monthly at my worst to six monthly when I didn't feel too bad. Anne worked on me from a distance being based in Scotland, occasionally we would visit her and she would work with me in person. Her reports following healing sessions are amazing, shedding light on past lives and what energies I have needed to release from this life and previous ones. What became apparent was the fact that my work was not doing me any good in terms of my health. Being a sensitive soul it appeared that I was picking up a lot of negative energy from the damaged souls with whom I was working. In one of the later 'in person' sessions with Anne, she picked up cancer energy within me, but dealt with it at that time. Anne encouraged me to seek medical advice, subsequent tests failed to show anything at that time. I continued to work, continued to stress my body, Anne was fire fighting each time she gave me some healing.

Things gradually began to go downhill, the itching was getting worse, my fungal nail infection was rapidly spreading. Coincidentally, an ex-colleague of Sandra's had been to see a naturopath by the name of Jan Ford-Batey, who held clinics locally. Jan's website www.naturetoheal.com describes her work thus:

> "By drawing on the very latest advances in conventional health sciences and research, and integrating them with a range of safe, effective natural therapies and age-old traditional medicines, Naturopathy or Naturopathic Medicine offers a truly holistic way of assessing, preventing and treating conditions of both the body and the mind.
>
> Whilst taking into account all aspects of current state of wellbeing - physical, mental and emotional - Naturopathic Medicine not only provides symptomatic relief, but also seeks to address the underlying causes of illness and disease, in a supportive rather than suppressive manner."

The ex-colleague of Sandra's had been cured of the fungal nail infection. I was, by now in a state. I booked an appointment and went to see Jan. She carried out muscle testing (kinesiology) to determine where my body was at. She was worried with what she found. At a cellular level, things were pretty bleak to say the least, my cells were on the verge of collapse. Jan suggested a high protein diet, including meat if I could tolerate it, but I had to avoid sugar, yeast and any foodstuffs potentially containing fungus, the same diet as for persons suffering with Candida. In addition I was given a number of supplements to aid my system and to counteract the huge fungal infestation that my body was experiencing. For my emotional side she suggested a number of approaches to help. The first of these was a process involving tapping the energetic meridians of the body known as Emotional Freedom Technique (EFT). Along with this she recommended a spiritual healer by the name of Ray Balmain who was based in Newcastle. I began to see Ray on a monthly basis. He is an amazing healer who was able to give me an insight into the bigger picture, in terms of my spiritual journey.

Jan also suggested various Bach flower remedies to give me emotional support depending upon how I was whenever she tested me. An occasional detoxification programme, especially for my liver, was another important facet of Jan's work with me. Jan tested my adrenal system through use of a private laboratory which used saliva tests to diagnose 'adrenal exhaustion'. The report was as follows:-

> "Exhaustion Stage: This is generally a state of insufficient production of adrenal hormones after multiple years of persistent stressors with insufficient coping mechanisms. Patients usually present with fatigue, poor energy and immune system hypofunction. They may exhibit chronic anxiety. In some patients this represents impaired response to short term stressors (i.e. over reactivity to short term stress). Adrenal support and restoration measures, as well as identification and balancing of major stressors are indicated."

That pretty well summed me up, my adrenal system was waving the white flag. It had had enough.

With all this support though, things gradually began to improve the itching was lessening and my nails were starting to return on my hands. Those on my feet, which had been like that for nearly thirty years, obviously took longer.

During my chemotherapy treatments I was aided with homeopathic remedies to help with the nausea and received much distance healing from Ray and Anne. I basically accepted whatever was given with gratitude. Since I finished treatment I have been seeing Jan on a regular basis and have been taking supplements to help support my body to recover and to cleanse itself of the toxic poisons that are chemotherapy, once they had done their job. I also took remedies with anti-cancer properties such as Essiac Tea and apricot kernels. Other immune boosters included included Life Mel™ and Manuka honey along with the likes of Alfalfa tonic. My immune system was under scrutiny and dietary advice along with initial dietary supplements helped to get my immune system back and working, recovering quicker than normal under such circumstances.

Finally, I have been seeing a Bio-Energy healer by the name of Briony Stott, this at the suggestion of Jan, who, on testing me last suggested that there were still some old emotional patterns that appeared to be holding me back from taking the final step to perfect balance. Briony describes herself as an 'energy cleaner' and sees her role as removing old energies from this and/or past lifetimes with a view to enabling the body to reach a balanced state. After a number of sessions it became apparent that I was carrying around a vast amount of stuck energies from this and past lifetimes which meant that the leukaemia was almost inevitable. Given the fact that Anne had already moved lots of such energies from me it is amazing to think I was upright and breathing carrying all this 'stuff' around with me!

My past lives have seen me as 'Essentially a man of peace' according to Briony but have, unfortunately included me being on the receiving end of much violence ! Anne has further found the fact that I have been carrying around lots of emotional energy. My past lives have included periods in slavery, being a monk, a knight of the Knights Templar and a child sweep in Victorian times among others. Being relieved of all this 'stuff' has placed me in a position in my life where I can now monitor my own energy field. I can now feel what is happening on an energetic level, feel what effect interactions with others has on me at an energetic level and respond accordingly. Now, for the first time in my life, I am in a position to balance myself as soon as imbalance occurs. It feels good I have to say. I do not take on the energies of others as I have in the past. I look forward to developing my spiritual practices and skills.

In addition I have made significant lifestyle changes. My diet has changed. Due to the cost of organic foodstuffs we rely on a product called 'Veggi Wash™' which is produced to rid vegetables and fruit of unwelcome chemical residues from pesticides etc. We have purchased a juicer and use this on a regular basis, juicing various fruit and vegetables. My diet consists of dairy produce, occasional bread, cereals, fruit, vegetables, pulses and occasional fish. We supplement this with nuts, seeds, dried fruit and the odd cake, biscuit or piece of chocolate !

We have installed a device in the house to combat geopathic stress which now appears to be working well. Water filters for the incoming water supply are the next purchase when funds will allow We already use water filters for our drinking water. Future plans include seeing Lorna the Medium for a psychic reading. We have seen Lorna a number of times in the past and she has always proved very accurate (even picking up the fact that cancer was on the horizon) and her skills can be used in order to get guidance from the higher realms to ensure that my spiritual journey continues to the benefit of all.

So, you can see that I have had a quite varied and intensive input from the complementary and alternative scene. The scientific fraternity would find evaluating how these have impacted on me difficult, and so tends to dismiss them. Nevertheless, the combination that I utilised was obviously to the benefit of my good self. I am still here, and a more balanced, grounded, stronger person for it. I am now in a position to move forward with my life and undertake and hopefully complete the mission I incarnated to achieve, with much mirth and joy along the way! Watch me begin to fly.....

Therapies & Remedies Galore!

It has been difficult to know how to lay out all the therapies that exist besides the traditional chemotherapy and radiotherapy, that is how to categorise them. Please bear with me as there are often overlaps, these are loose categories and are designed to give you a flavour as to what the therapies and remedies are about. There are ones I have left out, not deliberately but mainly because the idea behind this section is to give you some insight into the wealth of choice that you have. Again, I reiterate the fact that I am not giving you advice on which therapies to use, who am I to tell you what to do, choosing is a part of your own journey. Whatever you decide through your own intuition will be right for you.

- **Clinically Based Therapies**

    - Hormone Therapy
    - Hyperthermia (heat treatment)
    - Electrotherapy (ECT) or galvano therapy
    - Photodynamic cancer therapy (PDT)
    - Treatments with blood
        - Autohaemotherapy
        - Ozone-therapy, ozone-autohaemotherapy
        - Haematogenic oxidation-therapy (HOT)
- Biological Therapies
        - Immune stimulation with well-defined and effective drugs
        - Endogenous fever therapy with drugs such as interferon, interleukins   and bacterial derivatives
        - Active specific immune therapy ASI (vaccine to activate self-defense)
        - Dendritic vaccine

- Orthomolecular Medicine
- Vitamins, phyto nutrients, fatty acids, minerals, micro-nutrients, trace elements, amino acids and enzymes

- **Holistic Approaches**

  - Ayurvedic Medicine
  - Traditional Chinese Medicine (including massage, acupuncture etc)
  - Naturopathy

- **Natural Remedies / Herbal Medicine**

  - Phototherapy (medicinal plants)
    - Mistletoe therapy, phyto nutrients, Chinese herbs
  - Herbalism
  - Metabolic Therapy – Dr Hans Nieper
  - Essiac Herbal Tea
  - Vitamin B17 Metabolic Therapy
  - Graviola
  - Homeopathy

- **Detoxification**

  - Colonic Irrigation
  - Liver & Gall Bladder Cleansing
  - Hydro-colon therapy (intense intestine cleaning)
  - pH balancing

- Far infrared Sauna
- Direct current footbath (body check)
- Antioxidants (to detoxify from harmful metabolism waste products)
- Radical scavengers (to neutralize harmful free radicals)
- Intestinal ecology by probiotics
- Special nutritional and fasting programs
- Chelation therapy to eliminate toxins, carcinogens and heavy metals"

- **Energy Based Therapies**

  - Acupuncture
  - Bio-Energetic Healing
  - Sound Healing
  - Reiki
  - Crystal Healing
  - Reflexology
  - Chiropractic
  - Theta Healing
  - Spiritual Healing

- **Miscellaneous 'Hands On' Therapies**

  - Massage
    - Lymphatic Drainage
    - Swedish
    - Hot Stone
    - Deep Tissue

- Indian Head
- Bowen Therapy
- Alexander Technique
- Aromatherapy
- Acupressure
- Hellerwork

- **Psychological Therapies**

  - Counselling
  - Cognitive Behavioural Therapy
  - Psychotherapy
  - Past Life Regression

- **Emotional Clearing Techniques**

  - Emotional Freedom Technique (EFT)
  - Bach Flower Remedies
  - The Journey™
  - Hypnotherapy

- **Stress Busters**

  - Prayer
  - Meditation
  - Yoga
  - Tai Chi
  - QiQong
  - Exercise
  - Sleep

- Regular Mealtimes

- **Immune System Boosters**

  - Life Mel Honey™/ Manuka Honey
  - Alfalfa Tonic
  - Echinacea
  - Beta-Glucan
  - Ginseng
  - Sunlight Exposure – Vitamin D

- **Miscellaneous Aids**

  - Water Purification Filters
  - Devices to combat Geopathic Stress

This list is by no means exhaustive and no doubt there will be some therapists somewhere hopping about in a rage as I failed to include their therapy! Also I do not intend to go on and describe each therapy or remedy as there would be enough information to fill a book, indeed whole books have been dedicated to individual therapies! If you are interested in a particular therapy or remedy we are blessed to live in an age where information is at our fingertips, so happy searching !

The Cancer Diet – Fact or Fiction ?

To lead a healthy lifestyle is not cheap – fact. To buy organic food and eat lots of fresh fruit and vegetables comes at a price. Until there is a culturally driven change to alter this fact, we will be put in the difficult position of trying to fund our own healthy way of being. The more of us do this, however, the greater the drive for change. We are reminded that about a quarter of all cancer deaths are thought to be caused through unhealthy diets and obesity. Cancer Research UK have stated that our diet influences many cancers such as those of the bowel, stomach, mouth and breast. It is widely accepted that a balanced diet high in fibre, fruit and vegetables while being low in red and processed meat, saturated fat and salt is of benefit to us health wise.

There is much conflicting advice for the cancer sufferer with regard to dietary intake. What is noticeable is the lack of dietary advice from orthodox medicine, from personal experience the 'cram the calories' professional advice following chemo was hardly evidence based and scientific. I shall give two examples of dietary advice for the cancer sufferer. Dr Hans Nieper suggests in his book *'Dr Nieper's Revolution in Technology Medicine and Society'* that the following foods should be avoided:-

- No meat and no sausage. (In the case of exhaustion, lack of blood protein, or cachexia, very little meat- six or seven ounces per week)
- Little cheese
- Very little sugar
- Very little fast releasing carbohydrates, such as pastries and puddings
- No shellfish because of high nuclein content
- No smoking
- Very little alcohol

- No "junk" beverages
- No apple juice (too rich in glucose)
- No distilled water

While foods to be preferred are as follows:-

- Oat meal, millet, whole grain bread
- Skimmed milk
- Fish in limited quantity
- Fruit and fibrous vegetables, cooked and raw
- Carrot juice
- Pancraetic enzyme preparation
- Omniflora preparations, 'Eupalan' bifidum flora containing milk

Andreas Moritz has the following to say about diet and cancer:

" Eating a balanced vegetarian diet is one of the most effective ways to prevent cancer. If you feel you cannot solely live on foods that are of vegetable origin, then at least try to substitute chicken, rabbit or turkey for red meat for a period of time....All forms of animal protein decrease the solubility of bile, which is the major risk factor for developing gallstones, as well as lymph and blood vessel wall congestion. These are the main causes of cell mutation, which lead to cancer"

Additionally, it is widely recognised that cancer feeds on sugar. The metabolism of malignant tumours is largely dependent upon glucose consumption. It is a fact that insulin production triggers inflammation. Surely patients with tumours should be made aware of this at least, giving the tumour sufferer advice to go and cram the calories (which implies eating sweet foods and carbohydrates in particular) is bad advice in this context.

So, are you confused? I have to admit that I was debating whether to include a section on diet due to all the conflicting advice. However, we all have an innate wisdom within us which knows what is best for us at a particular time. For me, the cravings of meat were an attempt by my body to get protein. It is also noticeable that as things have settled down my incredibly sweet tooth has gone. A square of chocolate now suffices as opposed to the whole bar and some more in the past. My naturopath, Jan, was full of sensible common sense advice and worked with me monitoring my body and immune system, particularly focusing upon and building up the latter with natural supplements. Whatever works to get you through chemo then follow your nose, so to speak. It may be prudent at a later stage to examine your diet having gathered more information for yourself on the subject. The aim then surely has to be establishing a healthy and balanced regime for the future. When you later reflect on your dietary intake post cancer, it may well be that your revised diet is not far from what certain people have been advocating!

Cross my Palm with Silver...

In the UK as we have seen, the NHS does not offer us the luxury of a choice of treatments it tends to be the old double act of chemotherapy and his much maligned side kick radiotherapy. That leaves the likes of you and me in a bit of a financial dilemma. In order to tap into this vast array of potentially healing therapies and remedies we have to pay for it. Often when cancer strikes, there is an increased financial burden in any case due to a reduced income. Even where private health care policies exist, these do not generally include access to complementary medicine, and where they do it tends to be through referral from an orthodox medical practitioner, and for small amounts. Despite all these obstacles, we are still spending over £3 billion annually on complementary therapies and observing the complementary therapies market increasing annually at between 10 and 15 per cent irrespective of economic depression. Surely someone in so called authority has to take notice of this fact soon......

At the end of the day we have a hard decision to make that involves how strongly we believe in something. It may well be that financial circumstances dictate your decision and means that you have to solely rely on what is offered through the NHS, which it has to be said is somewhat restrictive. Actually spending money on ourselves is a major signal that we are taking responsibility for our own health. There are, it has to be said, cheaper alternatives available such as a pot of immune boosting honey, every little helps. It is unfortunate that a number of people leave approaching complementary and alternative therapists until they have run out of hope elsewhere and this is the last resort. In such circumstances the body may often be beyond repair. Maybe if we had taken action when the first warning lights came on then we possibly could have avoided the aftermath or at least lessen its impact. The bottom line is YOU ARE WORTH IT !!

Chapter Twelve

A Simple Man's Model of How to Approach Cancer

The Model

This is given in good faith for the benefit of others. It is given as my view gained through personal experience, use your own discernment (your heart) to determine whether it is for you. No psychobabble, no theories studies or surveys, as I see it just plain old common sense........

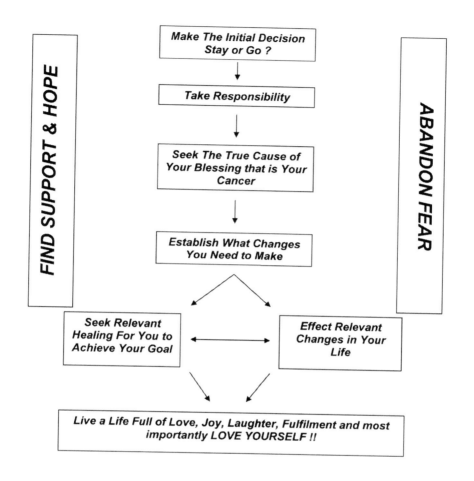

This model is given to you with hope that it will serve you in a way that will enrich your life and lead you to blossom and fulfil your vast potential that all we humans carry in us. It is formulated from the benefit of my own experience and from my knowledge up to this point in my life. I am not a guru, far from it and thus I am not in a position to tell anyone what they should or shouldn't do. It is given to you as a potential guide to assist you on your journey.

Make The Initial Decision.

Sounds so simple doesn't it, it may be a hard choice but to me, logically it is something that needs to be addressed. Without actually declaring to yourself that you intend to choose life, how else does your body know how to respond. It will just carry on doing as it always had. By making the decision to stay you will automatically set out your commitment and in so doing allow for change to occur. If you decide to leave this life, do so with the conviction that all will be well, death is not final, merely a stepping stone along the eternal journey that our souls are on. It can be a beautiful and peaceful experience if we allow it to be. It may be of benefit to talk through this process with loved ones, or if this is difficult, someone whom you respect and trust.

Fear, Hope and Support

Throughout the cancer journey it is important that you attempt to limit fear and stress (which are essentially the same thing, both bad for us in this scenario). As has been shown stress can inhibit any treatments we receive. There are numerous therapies which can help with this and having a good support network is also key to assisting you through.

I have heard it said that fear is an emotion we experience that is born of ignorance. Strong words, but what I think was meant was the fact that when we don't understand something or do not have full knowledge about a thing, that can lead us into the fear state. The more I found out about my condition (on all levels), the more my fear diminished. The other major fear that we seem to have is of the bloke with the cloak and scythe. Death is not something to be feared. We are immortal souls born of consciousness; we cannot die but live on in another form once we shed the bubble of biology that we have been custodian of from our entry into this beautiful world. Don't just take my word for it, look at what has been discovered through research into the subject. Knowledge can be a wonderful tool in tackling this fear monster that seems to follow us around.

It is important to remember though that there are many cases where those loved ones closest to us are often as terrified as we the cancer person are. It may be that support for the supporters is also required, and there are many wonderful, and often underused, support groups for exactly this situation. Most important is hope for the future. I found mine knowing that we are eternal spiritual beings and that no matter what happened I would be looked after. Maybe this is a time for you to examine your own belief system. However you do it, having hope is a vital component in the healing process. After all, without it why bother ?

Take Responsibility

This again sounds so easy, but when you consider that the current system (some call it 'The Nanny State') makes it the norm for us to rely on that system and to surrender our power to it, including our own health, it appears inevitable. The 'Victim Role' is almost welcomed by the state. We are responsible for our own bodies, our actions, thoughts, feelings and behaviours, if anyone tells you otherwise they are not serving your best interests. It is so hard for us to break away from this victim type philosophy because we are brought up with this belief that someone else, be it government, doctors and the like know what is best for us. Excuse me, where it is a matter of life and death I think I have the right to have just a wee bit to say on the subject! Given that you have chosen to stay, which would be nice as I can see you are a kindly soul, whichever course of action you choose, please do it from an informed standpoint, don't just roll over and give your power away.

Seek the True Cause of the Blessing that is Your Cancer

> " He who finds a purpose and meaning to the cancer within him will also find a way of curing it " Andreas Moritz.

Do not be deflated at this point and think that you are on your own with this one. For a start the above should fill you with hope and, as the old adage goes, 'Seek and ye shall find'. There are individuals out there who look at the body in a truly holistic way and can thus give you an insight into what is occurring to bring the blessing that is this cancer thing to you. I was blessed to find a Naturopath who utilised kinesiology as a diagnostic tool to determine where my body was and what was needed to rectify it as has been highlighted above. Traditional Chinese Medicine and Ayurvedic Medicine are systems that include a number of therapies and remedies along with potential lifestyle changes, both, however, will involve an initial assessment and subsequent diagnosis of your whole body. When was the last time an orthodox medical practitioner stated that the cause of your cancer was emotional blockages ? For spiritual guidance, again there are numerous practitioners out there who will be able to give you the big picture as to why you find yourself where you are today. You owe it to yourself to seek the cause, only then will true healing on all levels be allowed to begin.

Establish What Changes You Need to Make

When you begin to look after yourself it will become apparent what changes you need to make in terms of lifestyle changes. You may need to consider such aspects in your life as stress, smoking, alcohol intake, dietary intake, pollutants (such as toiletries, hair products, city living, water, food additives, pesticides etc), geopathic stress and exercise levels. You may need to look at your personality and effect changes that enable you to empower yourself and be more assertive. It may well be that you have emotional blockages from past trauma (who hasn't I hear you cry) that need healing. Finally, are you doing on the planet what you came here to do, or is it that your life has felt like a long search, from one relationship to the next, or one job to the next. Are you on the right spiritual path ? Do you find your life is full of joy, laughter and love ? If not it may be that you, like me need to evaluate what life is about, what ignites your passion and when you have found it, go do it.... and above all ENJOY IT!

The Final Steps....

In instigating the above and then finding healing through whatever method(s) you choose, you will probably be in a position to begin again. You will in all likelihood be a different person to the one who started out hearing those dreaded words 'You have Cancer.....'. A stronger more self aware person who has a lot to offer the world and a lot of living to do, especially in joy, laughter and love, which will ultimately nourish you and keep you healthy from top to toe and feed the trillion or so cells you have at this time. I can see your cells dancing from here..... Look in the mirror and what do you see. May I be so bold as suggest that reflected there is a beautiful soul who has had a difficult journey through this thing called life but who is now going forward with a spring in their step and an exciting new chapter in their life is unfolding................

Chapter Thirteen

Imagine A World.........

Creating Our Version of Heaven on Earth

If you were to be given a blank piece of paper and I asked you to design your own world, what would you put on it ? I hope it would include some of the following:-

- ○ Like a lottery winner, all my needs are met – I no longer have to worry about survival
- ○ I have enough food to eat, the food is nutritious and healthy
- ○ I have a nice place to live
- ○ I have clothes that keep me warm/dry/cool as I need
- ○ I feel a part of and am supported and nurtured by, my community
- ○ There is no ill health
- ○ There is no pollution, the air is clear and pure, likewise the water
- ○ I live in a state of blissful, joyful happiness
- ○ I gain passionate fulfilment every day in the knowledge that my contribution serves the highest good
- ○ There is peace throughout the land
- ○ There are no hidden agendas on the planet, all live in harmony and co-operate for the good of all, each person respects everyone else
- ○ All animals are treated with respect and dignity

- ○ Humans work in harmony with nature
- ○ All Children are loved, nurtured, and educated in such a way as to promote their gifts and talents

We find ourselves at this point in time at the cusp of major planetary change. What will happen, I hear you cry ? The answer, my friend, is blowing in the wind.... It is down to you and I to create what we really want. As human consciousness rises, so too does our ability to create and manifest our own reality. Currently we rely on others to make our version of reality for us, we watch the news and all the perceived problems 'out there' which worry us and put us in a state of fear and then cry out to those in charge 'please do something'. The solutions which miraculously appear are usually involved in eroding our freedom and power, often very subtly, under the guise of protecting us and keeping us safe. "We have nothing to fear but fear itself" as Franklin D. Roosevelt said. Go back to your sheet of paper with your vision of the world on it, take back your personal power and do your part to help create a vastly different and beautiful world. We owe it to ourselves and others.

Integrated Healthcare, the Stepping Stone to a New Way of Being

There is a growing body of opinion amongst spiritual commentators that in years to come we will have reached a level of consciousness which results in the whole population enjoying perfect health. That is indeed something for us to look forward to, but we are not there yet, some would say we appear to be heading in the opposite direction given the increase in the incidence of such diseases as cancer. However, if we are to tackle our health we need to begin to look at the body in a different way from the way we are currently taught. There are a minority of individuals and organisations seeking to promote the Integrated Healthcare model. One such is an Integrative Cancer Consultancy called 'Cancer Options' which was founded by and is now led by a Registered Nurse by the name of Patricia Peat. This organisation carries out private consultations for individuals to help them holistically through their cancer journey.

Another, somewhat larger organisation is that of The Prince's Foundation for Integrated Health which was founded in 1993 by HRH The Prince of Wales to promote integrated healthcare for all. The Foundation has a vision which:-

"Is of a society in which people are inspired and enabled, individually and collectively, to achieve optimal health and wellbeing."

Furthermore, they see society being supported in a truly holistic healthcare environment which encourages individuals to become empowered to make healthcare choices that lead to a better quality of life. The choices offered will make use of all appropriate therapeutic approaches, healthcare professionals and disciplines. Now this seems more like it and certainly gets my vote. The Foundation is involved in numerous projects that seek to reduce health inequalities. Judgements and decisions are based on reason and informed through evidence.

I have already referred to the charity CANCERactive which has a wealth of resources for individuals seeking information regarding cancer. Their website http://www.canceractive.com/ states that their aim is to:

> "lay out all the relevant information on cancer prevention, cancer treatment, cancer support and holistic care so that no one need die of ignorance".

It is unfortunate that it was only until writing this book did I discover this wealth of information. For a Cancer Centre of Excellence, such as I attended in Newcastle, not to give out such resources especially when individuals express an interest in complementary medicine is a fact I find both extraordinary and sad.

The next step, if I may be so bold, is to put these approaches into practice. Wouldn't it be marvellous to have an NHS treatment centre which offers a range of orthodox and complementary therapies and operates with a truly holistic philosophy. This, ladies and gentlemen, is not pioneering, ground breaking or heresy. Remember the German model of healthcare, especially the St George's Hospital and what they could offer patients. Here's to a rosy future in which holistic healthcare becomes the norm, and we laugh as we look back at what we used to do under the guise of 'health'.

Final Musings and a Prayer for the Future

Reflecting on what started out to be jottings while lying watching amazingly coloured chemotherapy drugs slowly infuse through my body to the finished book you have just read I am now in a position where I have come to the end. It has been a privilege to be able to have the time, the energy and the inclination to bring this to you. My deepest hope is that the content will help you and others to navigate the murky waters that are cancer, not in a state of fear but in a state of empowerment. You are an amazing person, a beautiful soul, look in the mirror and be proud of the soul inhabiting a bubble of biology at this time.

I do not want to be seen to be directing others on their journey, what I have presented here is information which can empower you to make an informed choice on your path from now on. If just one thing that you read resonated with you, touched a nerve, struck a chord and helped you in some way then this has been a job well done as far as I am concerned. I am far from becoming an enlightened being, and continue along the healing path slowly eradicating all those things that have kept my body out of balance for all these years. For that reason I would not be so presumptuous as to think I am in a position to lecture to anyone as to what you should and shouldn't do. I have endeavoured to give you the benefit of the knowledge I have gained through my cancer blessing. The model I have presented, in my belief system will provide you with a framework within which I make the bold suggestion that true healing may take place. This based on personal experience and from studying what other survivors have said. How that healing occurs is entirely up to yourself.

My next goal is to begin to explore the world of integrative healthcare, this with a view to helping in developing this model of health. Quite how and when is, perhaps, the next part of my journey. In addition I have to admit to being drawn to certain healing modalities, in particular working with energy. To train as a Naturopath may well also be on the agenda, who knows? May I thank you for taking time to read this and indeed congratulate you on the first steps towards health as by reading this you are clearly taking responsibility for yourself. The only advice I will give you is to follow your heart. May all your dreams become your reality.

To bring the book to a close I wanted to leave things on a positive note. This vision prayer is taken from Diana Cooper's book *'2012 and Beyond'*, on reading it I could not think of a more fitting way to end the book, let us all pray and thus ensure such a scenario comes to pass:-

"I have a vision where all people are at peace, fed and housed, every child is loved and educated to develop their talents, where the heart is more important than the head, and wisdom is revered over riches.

In this world justice, equality and fairness rule. Nature is honoured, so the waters flow pure and clear and the air is fresh and clean. Plants and trees are nurtured and all animals are respected and treated with kindness. Happiness and laughter prevail.

And humans walk hand in hand with angels. Thank you for the love, understanding, wisdom, courage and humility to do my part to spread the light. May all the world ascend. So be it."

References

Preface

Armstrong, Lance *It's Not About the Bike: My Journey Back to Life* Penguin US 2002

Chapter Four

Van Mil, J & Archer-Mackenzie, C *Healthy eating During Chemotherapy* Kyle Cathie Ltd London 2008

Chapter Seven

Becker, Harold W. *Unconditional Love - An Unlimited Way of Being* Florida US The Love Foundation 2008

Chopra, Dr Deepak *Quantum Healing : Exploring the Frontiers of Mind/Body Medicine* Bantam Books New York 1989

Cooper, Diana *Angel Answers* Hodder & Stoughton London 2007

Cooper, Diana *2012 and Beyond* Findhorn Press Forres Scotland 2009

Dongo,P & Raffill,T *China's Super Psychics* Da Capo Press Cambridge Mass. US 1997

Hodgkinson, Tom *How To Be Free* London Penguin 2007

Lipton, B *The Biology of Belief* Hay House Publishing London 2008

Melchizedek, Drunvalo *The Ancient Secrets of The Flower Of Life Volume One* Light Technology Arizona US 1998

Melchizedek, Drunvalo *The Ancient Secrets of The Flower Of Life Volume Two* Arizona US Light Technology 2000

McKenzie, Eleanor *Healing Reiki* London Hamlyn 2001

Tolstoy, Leo *The kingdom of God is Within You* London: OUP, 1936

Weiss, Dr Brian *Many Lives, Many Masters* London Piatkus 1988

Yogananda, Paramahansa *Autobiography of a Yogi* San Rafael USA Self-Realization Fellowship

http://www.drgaryschwartz.com

Chapter Eight

Abel, Dr Ulrich *Chemotherapy of Advanced Epithelial Cancer: A Critical Review* Journal of Biomedicine and Pharmacotherapy, 1992; 46: 439-452.

Goodman LS, Wintrobe MM, Dameshek W, Goodman MJ, Gilman A and McLennan MT. *Nitrogen mustard therapy. Use of methyl-bis(beta-chloroethyl)amine hydrochloride and tris(beta-chloroethyl)amine hydrochloride for Hodgkin's disease, lymphosarcoma, leukemia, and certain allied and miscellaneous disorders.* J Am Med Assoc 1946;105:475-476. Reprinted in JAMA 1984;251:2255-61.

Lipton, B *The Biology of Belief* Hay House Publishing London 2008

Moritz, Andreas *Cancer Is Not A Disease It's A Survival Mechanism* Llandeilo Cygnus Books 2009

Null, G et al *Death by Medicine* Nutrition Institute of America 2003 National Health Statistics Report Number 18 *Costs of Complementary and Alternative Medicine (CAM) and Frequency of Visits to CAM Practitioners United States, 2007*

Pal SK, Mittal B. *Improving cancer Care in India: Prospects and Challenges* Asian Pacific Journal of Cancer Prevention Jun;5(2): pp 226-8 2004

Starfield, B. *Is US Health Care Really the Best in the World ?* Journal of The American Medical Association July 26 284 (4) 483-485 2000

Thomas K, Coleman P, Nichol J; *Use and expenditure on complementary and alternative medicine in the UK. Annual Meeting of the International Society of Technological Assessment in Health Care Meeting.* 2002; 18: abstract no. 313.

Willett, W.C. *Balancing Life-Style and Genomics Research for Disease Prevention* Science 296: 695-698 2002

http://www.cancer.org The American Cancer Society – *Cancer Statistics 2008 Presentation*

http://www.who.int/en The World Health Organisation *World Health Organisation Statistics 2008.* 2009

http://www.who.int/en The World Health Organisation *World Cancer Report 2003*

http://www.freshminds.co.uk/PDF/THE%20REPORT.pdf

http://www.cancerbackup.org.uk

http://en.wikipedia.org/wiki/History_of_cancer_chemotherapy

http://www.cancer.org/downloads/AA/ACS_Combined_ Financials_FY2007.pdf

American Cancer Society Inc. & Affiliated Entities *Combined Financial Statements As of and for the Years Ended August 31 2007 and 2006*

http://annonc.oxfordjournals.org/cgi/content/full/mdl498v1   J Ferlay, P Autier, M Boniol, M Heanue, M Colombet and P Boyle *Estimates of the cancer incidence and mortality in Europe in 2006* Annals of Oncology published online on February 7, 2007

http://www.parliament.uk J Hicks and G. Allen Research Paper 99/11 *A century of Change: Trends in UK Statistics Since 1900* 21 December 1999

http://cancertrials.nci.nih.gov/cancertopics/factsheet/Therapy/gene#3

http://www.rccm.org.uk

http://www.nice.org.uk

http://www.ncri.org.uk

http://www.statistics.gov.uk/statbase/

http://cancernet.cicams.ac.cn

http://www.cancer.gov/cancertopics/factsheet/Therapy/biological

http://www.germancancertherapies.com

http://www.answers.com/topic/linus-pauling

Chapter Nine

Azar, B *Probing Links Between Stress & Cancer* American Psychological Association Journal 'Monitor' Vol 30 Issue 6 June 1999

Baines, C *Screening for Breast Cancer: How Useful Are Clinical Breast Examinations?* Journal of the National

Cancer Institute, Vol. 92, No. 12, 958-959, June 21, 2000

Brown, H.S. et al *The role of skin absorption as a route of exposure for volatile organic compounds (VOCs) in drinking water.* American Journal of Public Health 1984 Vol. 74, Issue 5 479-484

Bryson, Christopher *The Fluoride Deception* Seven Stories Press New York US 2004

Chopra, Dr Deepak *Quantum Healing : Exploring the Frontiers of Mind/Body Medicine* Bantam Books New York 1989

Ehrlich, A. *Building a sustainable food system.* In: Smith, P., ed. The world at the crossroads— Towards a sustainable, equitable and liveable world. London, Earthscan, 1994, p. 21-35.

Garland, C. Et al *Could Sunscreens Increase Melanoma?* American Journal of Public Health Vol. 82 No. 4 April 1992 614-615

Hansen, *J Light at Night, Shiftwork, and Breast Cancer Risk* Journal of the National Cancer Institute 2001 93: 1563 -1568

Halvorsen, Dr Richard *The Truth About Vaccines* Gibson Square Books London 2009

Heaney, R. *Vitamin D in Health and Disease* Clinical Journal Of American Nephrology 2008; 3 1535-1541

Heritage,J *The fate of Transgenes in the Human Gut* Nature Biotechnology 22(2) p 170+ 2004

International Food Policy Research Intitute (IFPRI). *A 2020 Vision for food, agriculture, and the environment.* Washington, D.C., IFPRI, 1995. p. 1-45.

Karpasea-Jones, J *Everything There is to Know about Vaccination* Meadow Books Cornwall 5th Ed 2006

Kulik, G. et al *Epinephrine Protects Cancer Cells from Apoptosisvia Activation of cAMP-dependent Protein Kinase and BAD Phosphorylation* The Journal of Biological Chemistry, May 11th 2007 (282) pp 14094-14100.

Lawrence, Felicity *Not On The Label* Penguin Books London 2004

Lipton, B *The Biology of Belief* Hay House Publishing London 2008

Mariea,T & Carlo G L *Wireless Radiation in the Etiology and Treatment of Autism: Clinical Observations and Mechanisms* Journal of the Australian College of Nutrition & the Environmental Medicine Vol. 26 No.2 (August 2007) pp 3-7

Miller, A et al *Canadian National Breast Screening Study-2: 13-Year Results of a Randomized Trial in Women Aged 50–59 Years* Journal of the National Cancer Institute, Vol. 92, No. 18, 1490-1499, September 20, 2000

Mingji, P. *Cancer Treatment with Fu Zheng Pei Ben Principle*,1992 Fujian Science and Technology Publishing House, Fujian.

Moritz, Andreas *Cancer Is Not A Disease It's A Survival Mechanism* Llandeilo Cygnus Books 2009

Netherwood,T. et al *Assessing the Survival of Transgenic Plant DNA in the Human Gastrointestinal Tract* Nature Biotechnology 22(2) p204+ 2004

Nieper, Hans *Revolution in Technology, Medicine and Society* MIT Oldenburg Germany 1981

Ott JN. Interview by Bland JS. American Journal of Preventative Med Update 1991; (Jan).Ott JN. Lecture to Society for Clinical Ecology, 1974.

Sadetzki, Dr S. et al *Cellular Phone Use and Risk of Benign and Malignant Parotid Gland Tumors—A Nationwide Case-Control Study* American Journal of Epidemiology 15 February 2008; 167: 457 - 467.

Serafini, M. Et al *This New Invention to Prolong Shelf Life* British Journal of Nutrition 2002   88: (6) pp 615-623

Weiss, Dr Brian *Many Lives, Many Masters* London Piatkus 1988

http://www.stress.org/uk

http://www.eatwell.gov.uk/healthydiet/eatwellplate/

http://www.eatwell.gov.uk/healthydiet/nutritionessentials/vitaminsandminerals/vitamind/

http://www.cancer.ca

http://www.co-operative.coop/food/ethics/Environmental-impact/Guide-to-pesticides/Banned-by-the-Co-op/

http://www.soilassociation.org

http://www.dailymail.co.uk/news/article-393666/Alarm-beef-link-breast-cancer.html

http://www.thefishsite.com/fishnews/9930/gm-salmon-ready-to-make-a-splash

http://www.rolfgordon.co.uk/

http://www.vegansociety.com/food/nutrition/vitaminD.php

http://www.vaccineriskawareness.com/

http://www.cancerhelp.org.uk/type/breast-cancer/about/screening/mammograms-in-breast-screening

http://www.cancerscreening.nhs.uk/breastscreen/publications/breastaware.pdf

http://www.anticancerinfo.co.uk

http://www.canceractive.com

http://www.independent.co.uk/news/uk/this-britain/tesco-hits-a-new-low-with-arrival-of-the-163199-chicken-778672.html

http://www.tastetech.co.uk

http://www.actionbioscience.org/biotech/sakko.html

http://www.foodnavigator.com/Product-Categories/Meat-fish-and-savoury-ingredients/Finnish-ministers-stir-up-GM-meat-debate

http://www.naturalnews.com/022630.html

http://www.healingdaily.com/detoxification-diet/soy.htm

http://www.infoforhealth.org/pr/m13/m13chap1_2.shtml

http://www.soyconnection.com/health_nutrition/index.php

http://www.second-opinions.co.uk/no-joy.html

http://www.healthyandwise.co.uk/geopathic.htm

http://www.leukaemia.org/what-we-do/campaigning/electricity-childhood-leukaemia

http://www.hpa.org.uk/HPA/Topics/Radiation/UnderstandingRadiation/1199451940308/

http://www.worldwithoutcancer.org.uk/

http://www.advisorybodies.doh.gov.uk/coc/drink.htm

http://www.water.org.uk/home/policy/positions/chlorine

http://www.who.int/foodsafety/publications/chem/acrylamide_faqs/en/index.html

http://www.codexalimentarius.net/web/index_en.jsp

http://www.therealessentials.com/sinistertruth.html

http://www.citizen.org/documents/codextoronto.pdf

Chapter 10

Bays, Brandon *The Journey* Harper Collins London 1999

Challis,G. & Stam, H. *The Spontaneous regression of Cancer : A Review of Cases from 1900 to 1987* Acta Oncologica 1990;29(5): pp545-50.

Chopra, Dr Deepak *Perfect Health: The Complete Mind/Body Guide* Bantam Books New York 1990

Cole WH, Everson TC: *Spontaneous Regression of Cancer.* WB Saunders, Philadelphia, US 1966

Hirshberg,C & O'Reagan B *Spontaneous Remission – An Annotated Bibliography* Institute of Noetic Sciences Petaluma US 1993

Hobohm,U. *Fever Therapy Revisited* British Journal of Cancer 92 pp421-425   Feb 2005

Moritz, Andreas *Cancer Is Not A Disease It's A Survival Mechanism* Llandeilo Cygnus Books 2009

Moseley, J. , O'Malley, K. et al *A Controlled Trial of Arthroscopic Surgery for Osteoarthritis of the Knee* New England Journal of Medicine 347(2) pp81-88 2002

http://www.noetic.org/research/sr/biblio.html

http://www.medterms.com/script/main/art. asp?articlekey=11287

Chapter 11

Brennan, Barbara H*ands of Light : A Guide to Healing Through the Human Energy Field* Bantam Books London 1988

Moritz, Andreas *Cancer Is Not A Disease It's A Survival Mechanism* Llandeilo Cygnus Books 2009

Nieper, Hans *Revolution in Technology, Medicine and Society* MIT Oldenburg Germany 1981

http://www.chopra.com/ayurveda
http://www.floweroflife.org
http://www.naturetoheal.com
http://www.worldbridger.biz/
http://www.rjbhealing.com/
http://www.brionystott.co.uk/

Chapter 12

Moritz, Andreas *Cancer Is Not A Disease It's A Survival Mechanism* Llandeilo Cygnus Books 2009

Chapter 13

Cooper, Diana *2012 and Beyond* Findhorn Press Forres Scotland 2009
http://www.canceroptions.co.uk/
http://www.fihealth.org.uk/
http://www.canceractive.com/

Lightning Source UK Ltd.
Milton Keynes UK
UKOW051905250112

186069UK00001B/61/P